SOLO's Field Guide
Wilderness
First Aid

Wilderness, Marine, Rural, Disaster, International

"Beyond the Golden Hour"

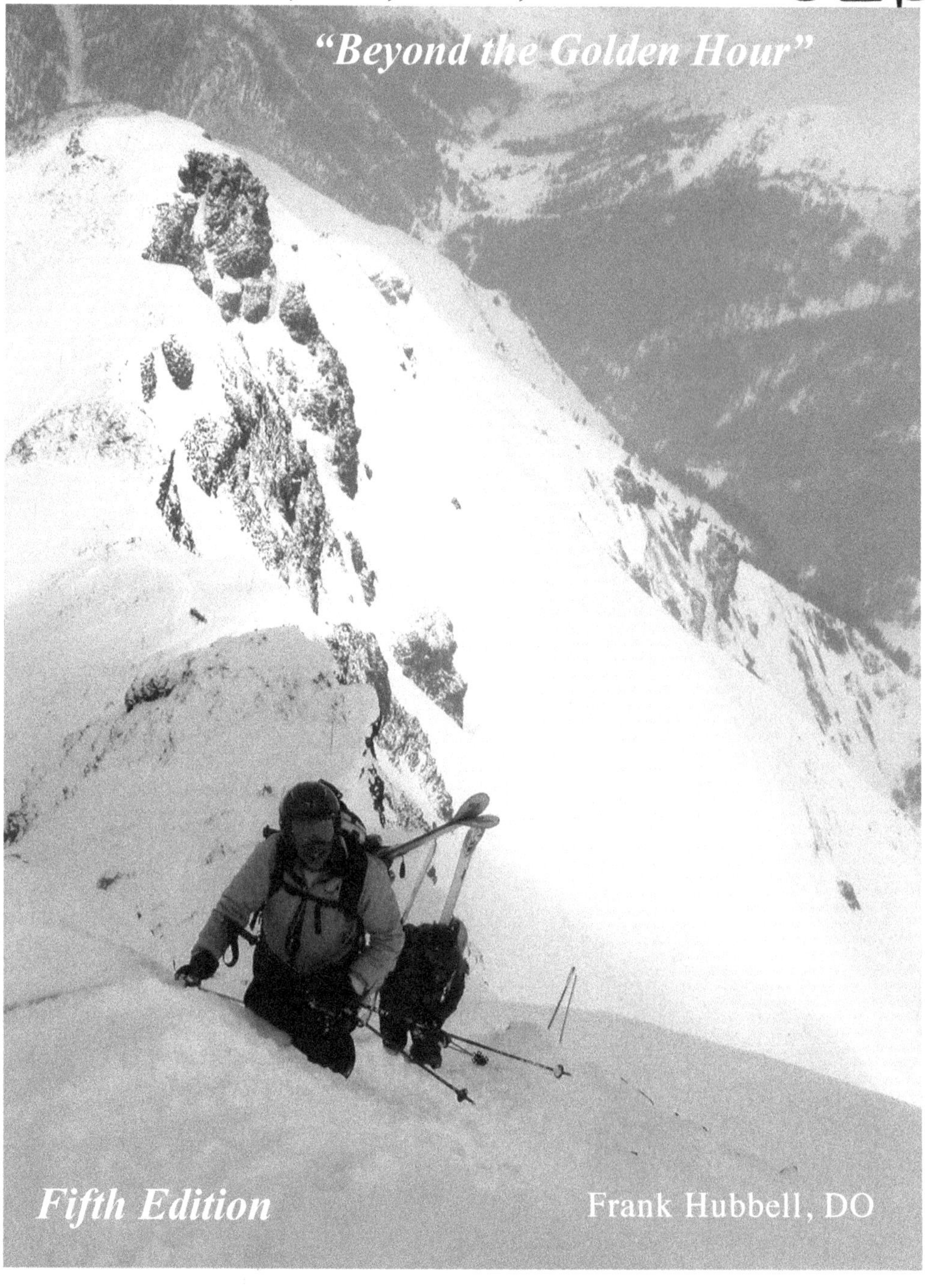

Fifth Edition

Frank Hubbell, DO

SOLO'S FIELD GUIDE TO WILDERNESS FIRST AID
FIFTH EDITION PAPERBACK

Published by:
TMC Books LLC
731 Tasker Hill Rd., Conway, NH 03818
info@TMCBooks.com
http://www.TMCbooks.com

ISBN: 978-1-7349308-6-3

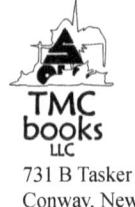

TMC
books
LLC
731 B Tasker Hill Rd.
Conway, New Hampshire
03818
U.S.A

This book is dedicated

to my co-founder, co-director, and wife, Lee Frizzell.

For without her heart, patience, and kind spirit, none of this would exist.

And to all the Good Samaritans who have the heart to stop and help.

Jesus replied and said, "A certain man was going down from Jerusalem to Jericho; and he fell among robbers, and they stripped him and beat him, and went off leaving him half dead.

"And by chance a certain priest was going down on that road, and when he saw him, he passed by on the other side.

"And likewise a Levite also, when he came to the place and saw him, passed by on the other side.

"But a certain Samaritan, who was on a journey, came upon him; and when he saw him, he felt compassion, and came to him, and bandaged up his wounds, pouring oil and wine on them; and he put him on his own beast, and brought him to an inn, and took care of him."

Luke 10:30-34
NAS

SOLO's Field Guide to Wilderness First Aid

The SOLO Field Guide to Wilderness First Aid is the manual that accompanies SOLO's two-day course of the same name. The Wilderness First Aid (WFA) course was created out of the direct experience of the founders of SOLO and is designed by and for the "outdoor enthusiast:" whether hiker, climber, skier, kayaker, canoeist, or sailor. It is for the adventurous who may find themselves away from immediate help and may have to rely on their own skills to survive and thrive if an emergency should arise.

First offered in 1974 under the name of the Mountain Rescue Seminar, the course next became Backcountry Medicine, and eventually Wilderness First Aid. The course has continued to evolve over the past 40 years, through over a thousand programs, and hundreds of thousands of students.

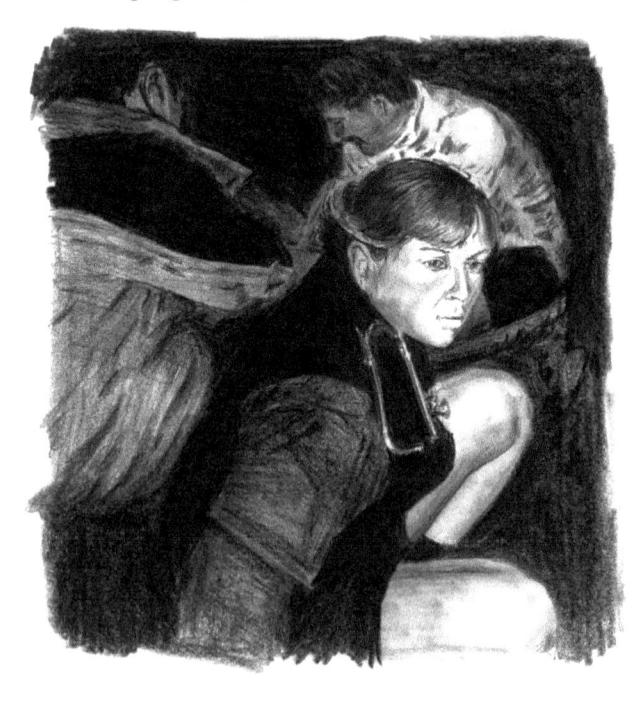

A jam-packed, fast-paced course, WFA covers a variety of topics including how to recognize and manage common medical problems along with rare but life-threatening emergencies, environmental emergencies, and most importantly, prevention of these problems. This textbook is intended to be a true field guide that our students can carry with them throughout their training with SOLO and use as a reference later.

This course is recognized by the American Camping Association as the minimal standard for camp counselors, both day hiking, and overnight hiking leaders. For professional outdoor leaders doing multi-day trips or expedition-level mountaineering, this course is a good start and will help prepare students for SOLO's Wilderness First Responder or Wilderness Emergency Medical Technician certification programs.

Table of Contents

Editor's Note: *We extend our apologies to grammarians for the often unorthodox use of punctuation marks and capital letters and for the intentional lack of agreement between pronouns and their antecedents.*

THE "WILDERNESS" IN WILDERNESS FIRST AID:

WHAT IS "WILDERNESS" AND WHY IS IT SO CHALLENGING TO THE EMERGENCY CAREGIVER?

In the world of pre-hospital medicine, the term "wilderness" or "extended care" is defined as any time a patient is more than an hour from definitive (hospital ER) care. The critical first hour after an injury occurs is called the "Golden Hour."

In the wilderness setting it is very easy to consume an hour in a rescue effort. When someone becomes sick or injured, a chain of events has to occur to get the patient out of the woods and into the hospital, and it is more than simply calling 911. Commonly, someone has to hike out and notify EMS; then EMS has to respond to the trailhead, hike back in to the patient, treat and package the patient, carry them out to the waiting ambulance, and finally transport them to the hospital. A general rule of thumb to estimate the total rescue time from injury to the hospital is one hour of effort for every quarter-mile from the road.

Distance and Time: it's farther and longer than you think.

- Rapid notification for help is usually impossible.
- Someone may have to go for help on foot. What information should they carry out?
- The response by the rescue team is prolonged; they usually have to walk in. What will you do until they arrive?
- Provision of emergency care is clearly outside the "Golden Hour."

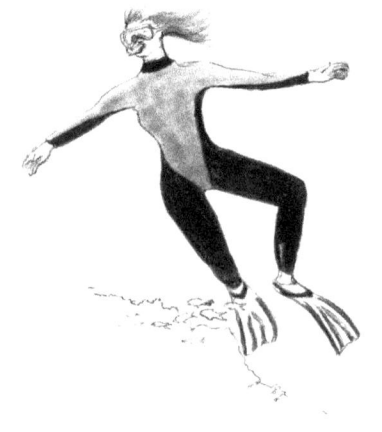

The Environment: can easily turn hostile.

- Cold, wet, snow, or darkness can delay rescuers even longer.
- Poor weather conditions can be a direct threat to the safety of rescuers, the patient, and others with the patient.
- Poor weather conditions may eliminate the possibility of access by helicopter.
- It can be much more difficult to take care of yourself, the patient, and anyone else on the scene.

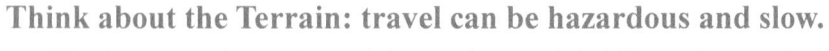

Think about the Terrain: travel can be hazardous and slow.

- Access to the patient might require special skills such as rock climbing ability or experience.
- Terrain features such as deep snow, deep mud, or even a steep trail can further slow rescuers.
- Terrain features may even present extreme dangers in the form of avalanches or flooded river crossings.
- There may be route-finding difficulties.

Equipment and Resources: maximize efficiency to minimize weight.

- Is the group to be rescued prepared for the conditions?
- Is the responding team "wilderness" trained and prepared for the conditions?
- The group must know how to improvise equipment.
- Limited equipment and access to resources is the norm.

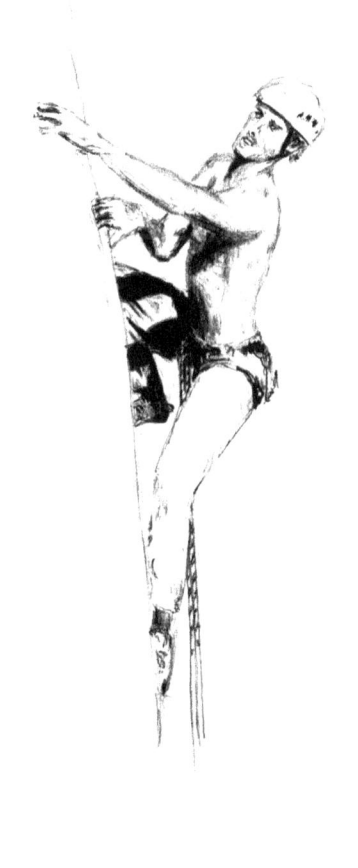

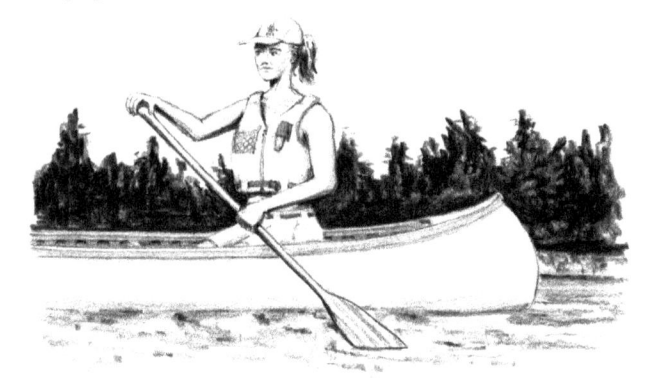

Specialized Training and Wilderness Knowledge: get smart.

- Map and compass and route-finding skills, search and rescue skills.
- Weather forecasting skills.
- Bivouac skills.
- Technical rescue skills, ropes and knots, water rescue skills.
- Understanding long-term patient care.
- Helicopter rescue training.

For all of these reasons wilderness care providers are expected to follow and to perform at a different standard of care than a care provider in an urban setting. As implied, someone learning wilderness first aid may need to learn and master a number of skills that are not directly related to patient care. They may also be expected to manage an injury differently than a caregiver in an urban environment simply because the wilderness care provider may be staying with the patient for a long time while waiting for help to arrive, and possibly while the patient is being transported to definitive care.

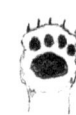

CHAPTER ONE

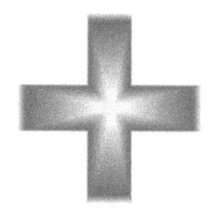

RESPONSE AND ASSESSMENT

What happened?

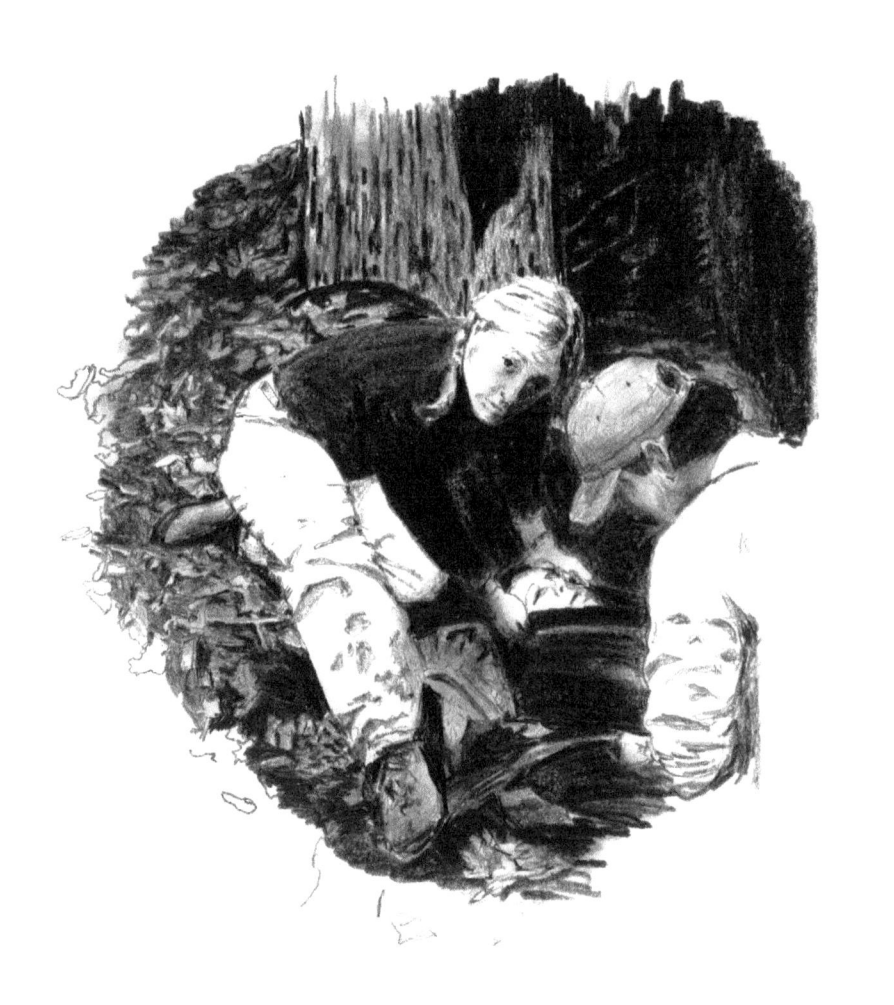

BODY SUBSTANCE ISOLATION (BSI):

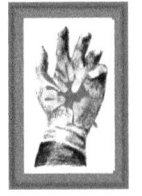

Also referred to as Total Fluid Precautions or Universal Precautions

In providing emergency medical care you can be exposed to infectious disease agents, and you need to know how to protect yourself against these disease-causing organisms.

Modes of Transmission

DIRECT CONTACT

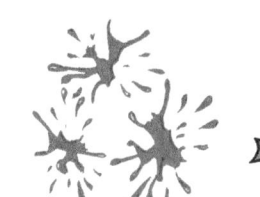

The spread of disease by direct contact with the blood or other body substances of an infected individual (saliva, sputum, blood, urine, feces, secretions).

INDIRECT CONTACT

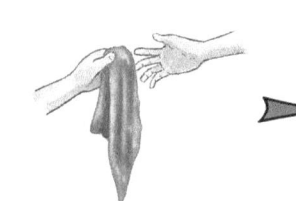

The spread of disease from one individual to another by touching a contaminated inanimate object (door knob, clothing, stretcher, countertop, etc.) and then transferring the pathogen to mouth or eyes with the now contaminated hands.

AIRBORNE

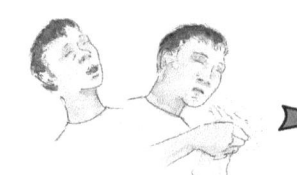

The spread of disease by infected droplets of saliva or sputum expelled into the air by coughing or sneezing and then being inhaled by another person.

VECTOR

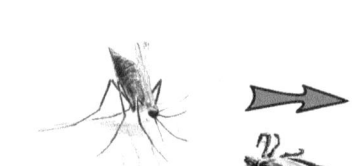

The spread of disease by blood-sucking insects, such as mosquitoes, fleas, or ticks.

WATERBORNE

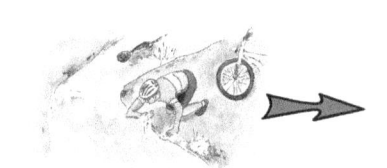

The spread of disease by the consumption of contaminated water, usually contaminated with human waste, the "oral fecal route."

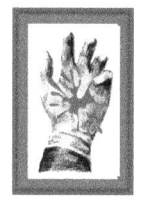

Our primary defense is behavior: we take precautions to prevent contamination. PREVENTION equals BEHAVIOR.

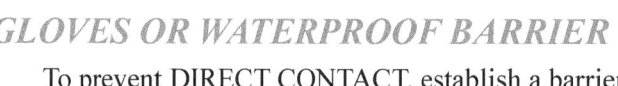

GLOVES OR WATERPROOF BARRIER

To prevent DIRECT CONTACT, establish a barrier before any potential exposure to body fluids.

HAND-WASHING

To prevent patient-to-patient and hand-to-mouth transfer of pathogens by INDIRECT CONTACT, wash hands before and after any patient contact.

MASKS

To prevent AIRBORNE spread, put on a surgical mask before any potential exposure to airborne pathogens, especially tuberculosis (put a mask on the patient, too, if possible).

INSECT REPELLENT, MOSQUITO NETTING, CLOTHING

To prevent the transmission of disease by blood-sucking insects, use insect repellents (Permethrin), wear protective clothing, sleep under mosquito netting, and do tick checks.

WATER PURIFICATION

To prevent waterborne illnesses always make and drink potable water by boiling, use of water filters, chemicals (iodine or chlorine), or the use of UVC light (Steripen).

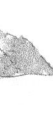
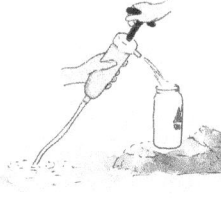

THE ANATOMY OF A CRISIS: THE PATIENT ASSESSMENT SYSTEM

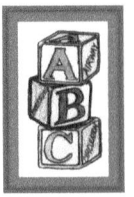

*These two pages are a quick overview of what to do if you come upon an accident scene. We will go over each of these four steps in much more detail but this is the **BIG** picture.*

What would you do if you were hiking along and were the first one to arrive at the scene of an accident?
- How would you find out what is wrong and what has happened?
- How do you tell how badly hurt the injured person is?
- Do you go for help?
- Do you try to help the injured person?
- What should you do?

The method used is STOP and Survey referred to as *The Patient Assessment System* which consists of a list of questions and tasks that need to be performed in order to ascertain what happened and what you are going to do about it.
- These questions and tasks are arranged by priority and should be done in order.
- You should not move on to the next task until the one you are on has been successfully completed.

FIRST—STOP—SCENE SURVEY: Is the scene safe?
- Are you safe? BSI?
- Is everyone else safe?
- Is the patient safe?
- What happened? (Mechanism of Injury—MOI)
- How do you safely approach the victim?
- What is your general impression of the situation's seriousness?

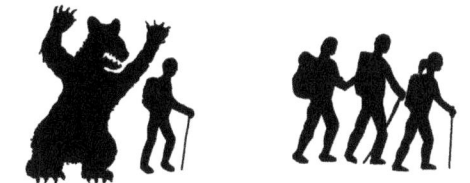

This first step is critical, to rush in before you have the whole picture might lead to a second accident.

Survey the scene!

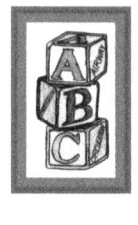

SECOND—STOP—Do a PRIMARY SURVEY: Are they alive?
Are there any life threats? The A B Cs...

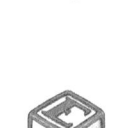

Approach, Assess, Airway—Are they conscious and can they speak?
—Do they have an open airway?

Breathing—Are they breathing? —How well are they breathing?

Circulation—Do they have a pulse? —Are they bleeding?

Deformity—Are there any obvious deformities?
—Is their neck or back at risk of injury?

Environment—Can they stay where they are?
—Is anyone else in the group at risk?

THIRD—STOP—Do a SECONDARY SURVEY: How Are They?

- What happened?—the History of Present Illness
- How well are they doing?—Vital Signs
- What are their injuries?—Patient Exam
- What is their past medical history?—**AMPLE** History
- What is your patient care plan? —**SOAPnote**

FOURTH—STOP—Do a RESCUE SURVEY: Do you need help?

- What is your plan to get help?
- Who is being sent for help?
- What do you need to do to protect the patient while waiting for help to arrive?
- What do you need to do to protect yourselves while waiting for help to arrive?
- Is the scene safe for the group?
- Perform on-going assessment; re-SOAP every 15 minutes.

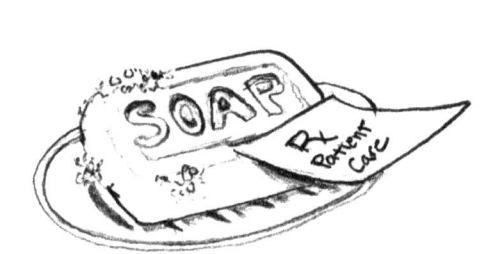

PATIENT ASSESSMENT SYSTEM IN DETAIL

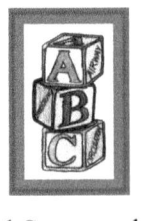

To survey something is to examine it closely and ascertain its condition. In this system of STOP and Survey, the intent is to take the time to STOP and take a deep breath before closely examining and ascertaining the patient's condition. A survey is organized in a logical step-by-step process that allows you to gather the information and respond in an orderly manner.

FIRST: STOP—SCENE SURVEY: Is the Scene Safe?

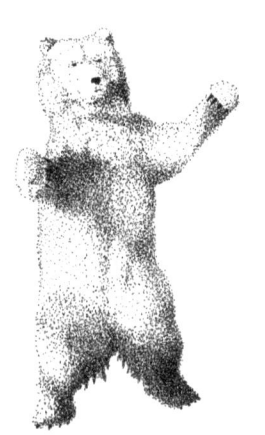

- Are you OK, and are you going to stay OK?
- Are the others OK, and are they going to stay OK?
- Is the victim of this crisis OK, and are they going to stay OK?
- What happened? What was the mechanism of injury (MOI)?
- How do you safely approach the victim?
- What is your general impression of how serious this is?

To accomplish all this Scene Survey:

Stop. Stand still, take a deep breath, and ask yourself, "Am I OK?" If not, do something about it! Go.

Stop. Tell everyone else to STOP, stand still, take a deep breath and ask themselves, "Am I OK?" If not, do something about it! Don't allow anyone to run off to check the victim or to get help. Go.

Stop. Is the victim OK? First speak or call out to them, even if you cannot see them or get to them. Ask them if they are all right. Hopefully, they will answer; even if they say that they are not all right, at least you know they are alive, have an open airway, are breathing, and have a pulse. Go.

Stop. Ask yourself, "What happened?" "What was the mechanism of injury?" Go.

Stop. Survey the victim's situation. While figuring out how to safely get to them, keep talking to them. Be positive, keep encouraging them, tell them to lie still, that help is on the way. Go.

Stop. As you approach the victim, survey their position. Ask yourself, "Can they stay where they are, or are they in imminent danger and need to be moved?" Go.

Stop. What is your impression of the victim? As you approach the victim (they do not become your patient until you lay your hands on them), develop a general impression of how serious the situation seems to be, based on the position they are lying in, how they look, whether they are conscious, bleeding, etc. Go.

SECOND: STOP—PRIMARY SURVEY:
Are they alive, and are they going to stay alive?

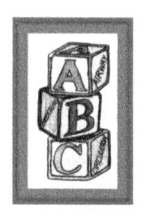

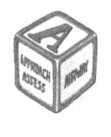 **Approach, Assess, Airway**—Is the victim conscious and can they speak?
—Do they have an open airway?

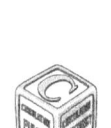 **Breathing**—Are they breathing? —How well are they breathing?

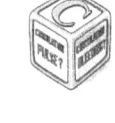 **Circulation**—Do they have a pulse? —Are they bleeding?

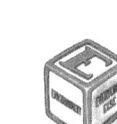 **Deformity**—Are there any obvious deformities? —Is their neck or back at risk of injury?

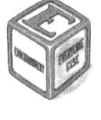 **Environment**—Can they stay where they are?
—How is everyone else in the group doing?

The PRIMARY SURVEY allows you to quickly assess how hurt or ill your patient is. You are looking for anything that might threaten the life of the patient, what we call "life threats". If you find a life threat, you need to stop and intervene, if you don't find any life threats, you can take a deep breath, and slow down because you have time.

- It also takes into consideration how the environment is impacting on the patient.
- If there is a problem, you do not move on to the next step until that problem is solved.
- Each aspect of the primary survey is explored by looking, listening, and feeling.

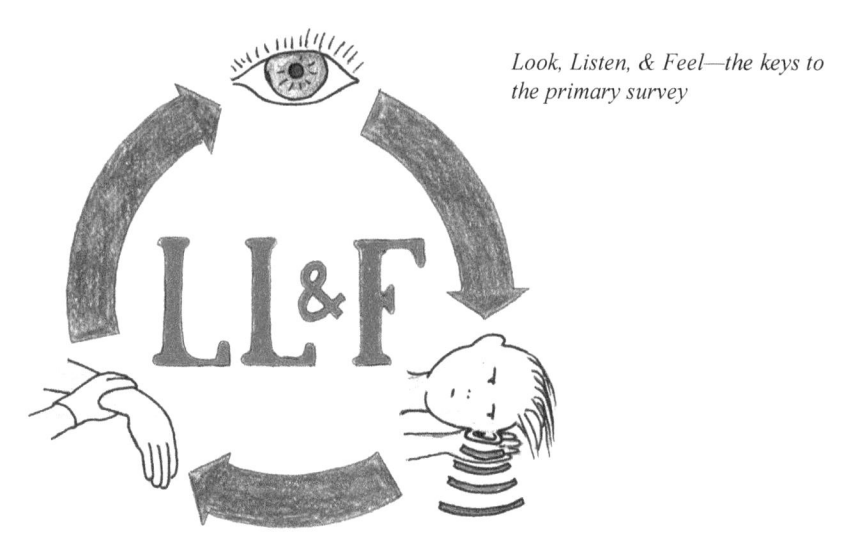

Look, Listen, & Feel—the keys to the primary survey

Now let's look at the ABCs in more detail...

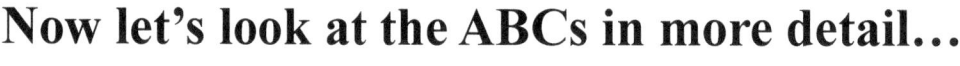 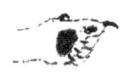

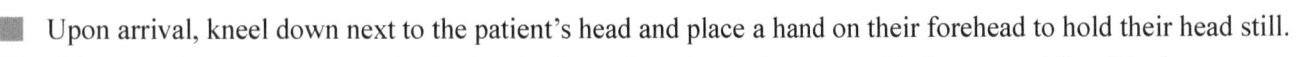

Approach and Assess—Are they conscious, and can they speak?

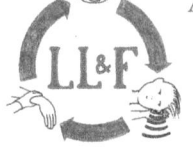

Look—Are they awake; are their eyes open; what position are they lying in?

Listen—Speak to them. Do they speak back?

Feel—What is your general impression of the situation?

◼ —If unconscious apply painful stimuli.

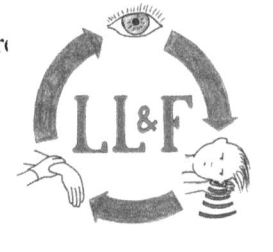
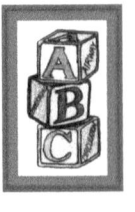

◼ Upon arrival, kneel down next to the patient's head and place a hand on their forehead to hold their head still.

◼ This not only protects the cervical spine, it also makes physical contact with them, providing "the human touch."

◼ Continue to speak to them even if they are unconscious.

◼ The first question you ask is are they conscious or unconscious? If they are conscious, can they speak?

◼ If they are conscious, ask them to lie still until you have had a chance to check them out.

◼ Ask the obvious questions: "Are you all right?" "Where does is hurt?" "Do you know what happened?"

◼ If they are unconscious, you need to make sure that they have an open airway.

To test for LOC, apply a painful, but harmless, stimulus.

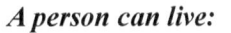

Airway—Do they have an open airway?

Look—Is there anything in their airway?

Listen—Can you hear air moving in and out of the airway?

Feel—Can you feel air moving in and out of the airway?

◼ Lean over your unconscious patient and place your ear in front of their mouth so that you can feel and hear air moving in and out of their airway.

◼ If they are not breathing, inspect the airway. The most common cause of an obstructed airway is the tongue and position of the head.

◼ To open the airway, move the head into proper anatomical position. Tilt it slightly back (extension), and gently pull the lower jaw (mandible) forward. This moves the musculature of the tongue forward and opens the airway.

◼ Again, place you ear over their mouth to make sure that they are breathing.

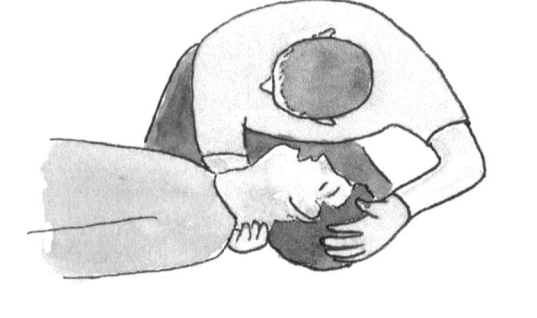

A person can live:

◼ Weeks without food.

◼ Days without water.

◼ Hours in a harsh environment without shelter.

◼ But only SIX MINUTES without oxygen.

Breathing—Are they breathing?

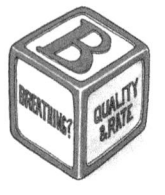

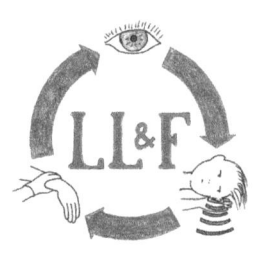

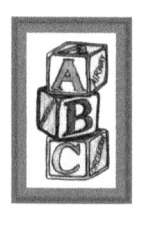

Look—Is their chest wall moving as they breathe?

Listen—Can you hear breath sounds?

Feel—Can you feel air moving in and out of their mouth?

- While leaning over, with your ear in front of their mouth, listen to them breathe and make sure air is moving in and out of the airway. Listen to their breath sounds.
- If they are not breathing, give them two full breaths and check to see if they have a pulse. If they have a pulse, continue to give them one full breath every 4–5 seconds until they are breathing on their own.
- If they do not have a pulse, initiate CPR.

Breathing—How well are they breathing?

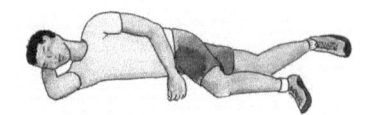

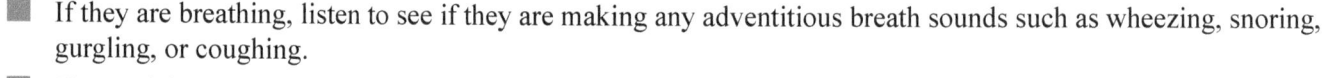

Look—What is their skin color (are they pale, ashen, blue)?

Listen—Can you hear any adventitious breath sounds such as wheezing, gurgling, or snoring, indicating a partially occluded airway?

Feel—Is the chest wall moving appropriately with respirations?

- If they are breathing, listen to see if they are making any adventitious breath sounds such as wheezing, snoring, gurgling, or coughing.
- If any of these sounds are heard, log roll the patient into the recovery position to help clear and maintain an open airway.
- In the recovery position gravity will drain any fluids from the airway and allow the tongue to fall forward opening the airway.
- Never tolerate any adventitious breath sounds as they indicate that the airway is at least partially occluded and the patient is not getting enough oxygen.
- Breathing includes not only whether they are breathing (is air moving in and out of the lungs), but also how well they are breathing.
- Are they breathing often enough and deeply enough to get an adequate supply of oxygen into the lungs and, therefore, into the blood.
- A normal respiratory rate is between 10–30 breaths per minute depending upon age and activity level.
- If they are not taking at least one breath every 6 seconds, 10 breaths per minute, then you need to assist ventilate with at least one full breath every 5–6 seconds.
- If their respiratory rate is greater than 1 breath every 2 seconds or 30 breaths per minute, they are breathing too fast and too shallowly to allow for good air exchange.
- Again assist ventilate them at a rate of one full breath every 5–6 seconds to improve the air exchange in the lungs.
- Now that you know they have an open airway and adequate breathing, check their pulse.

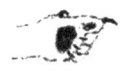

Circulation—Do they have a pulse?

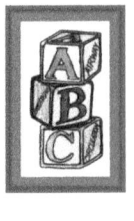
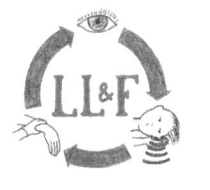

Look—Is their skin pale? Are they cyanotic (bluish)?
Listen—Can you hear a heartbeat?
Feel—Can you feel a carotid pulse?

- Once you have established that they have an open airway and they are breathing, check a carotid pulse.
- This is accomplished by placing your 2nd and 3rd fingers over the center of the trachea and drawing your hand towards yourself and into the groove between the trachea and the sternocleidomastoid muscles of the neck. As you gently compress this groove, you will be able to palpate the carotid artery pulse.

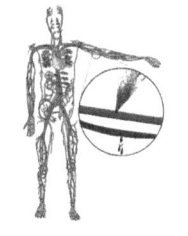

- If they do not have a pulse, initiate CPR. If for some reason you cannot access or feel the carotid pulse, you can place your ear over the left side of the chest to listen for a heartbeat.

Circulation—Are they bleeding?

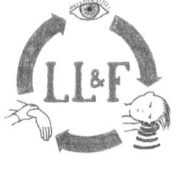

Look—Is there any active bleeding?
Listen—Can you hear a heartbeat?
Feel—Can you feel a carotid pulse?

- Along with determining if there is a pulse, you also need to scan the length of their body and look for any signs of obvious bleeding.
- If there are areas of blood in their clothing or blood pooling on the ground, inspect the area for any source of the bleeding.
- A minor scrape that is oozing blood can be ignored for now.
- Your concern is major bleeding from blood that is spurting from the body or rapidly flowing from a wound. This type of bleeding must be controlled.

Significant bleeding is a life threat!
You need to stop the bleeding before you go to the next step.

Stop the bleeding!

DIRECT PRESSURE

- Apply pressure directly to the wound with your gloved hand.
- If possible, place some absorbent material, such as gauze pads, on top of the wound before applying pressure—it will act as a sponge and help hold the blood in place.
- Because the vast majority of bleeding is venous, it is under low pressure, and can usually be controlled with gentle direct pressure.
  - It may take 10 – 20 minutes to completely stop the bleeding.
- Once the bleeding has stopped, maintain direct pressure for ten additional minutes to allow blood clots to form.

PRESSURE DRESSING

- If a wound bleeds stubbornly, or you need to do other things for your patient, you can apply a pressure dressing, which will maintain light pressure for you.

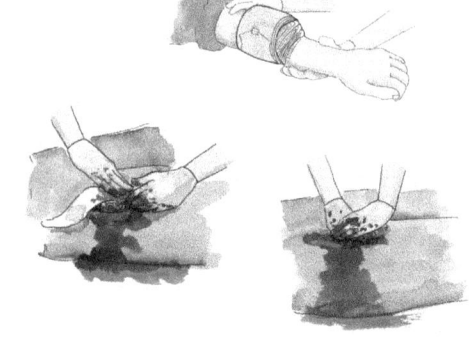

WOUND PACKING

- For a life-threatening bleed where a tourniquet can not be used, pack the wound with bleeding control gauze (hemostatic gauze), plain gauze, or a clean cloth and then apply pressure with both (gloved) hands.
- Apply steady pressure with both hands directly on top of the bleeding wound. Press down hard on the bleeding would and continue to press down.

TOURNIQUETS

If all your efforts to stop the bleeding fail, you may have to use a tourniquet and you've determined that the patient may die without it.

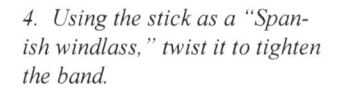

- A tourniquet is very rarely needed—do not apply it to simple wounds involving only venous bleeding; virtually all bleeding can be controlled with direct pressure and a pressure dressing. An example of a situation where a tourniquet may be needed would be a laceration of an artery (e.g., femoral or brachial) in a leg or arm.
- A tourniquet should only be used for extreme life-threatening arterial bleeding in an extremity that cannot be controlled any other way—for instance, if an arm or leg has been mangled or severed.
- Tourniquets are used on extremities only.

Improvised Tourniquet

1. Wrap a wide band around the extremity, not over clothing, at least 2" to 3" proximal to the bleeding and not over the elbow or knee.

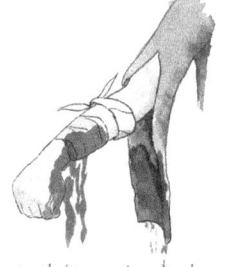

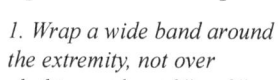

Locate the tourniquet above, or proximal, to the injury.

2. Tie a simple knot in the band.

3. Place a 6" stick or bar over the knot and tie a second knot over it to secure it.

4. Using the stick as a "Spanish windlass," twist it to tighten the band.

5. Tighten the windlass until both the bleeding and the distal pulse stop.

6. Secure the free end of the windlass in place with another band or tape.

7. Write a capital "T" and the time of application on the patient's forehead.

8. If possible, cold pack the extremity to increase the duration of survivability, just like an amputation.

9. Evacuate immediately.

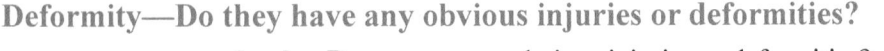

Deformity—Do they have any obvious injuries or deformities?

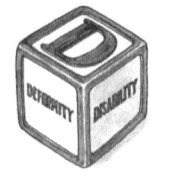

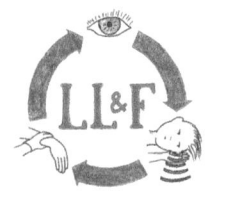

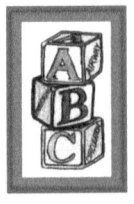

Look—Do you see any obvious injuries or deformities?

Listen—Where are they complaining of pain?

Feel—Where does it hurt? As you touch them, where can you cause pain?

- This is referred to as a "chunk check."
- Scan the length of the body looking for any obvious deformities like angulated fractures. See if there is anything sticking out of the body that belongs inside or anything sticking into the body that belongs outside.
- Then perform a chunk check by quickly palpating the major parts of the body.
- You want to gently compress the head, the neck, the chest, the abdomen, the pelvis, and the upper legs, feeling for injuries or pain response.
- If you find any injuries, take the time to inspect the area to see if there is something that you need to deal with immediately.

Disability—Is their neck or back at risk of injury?

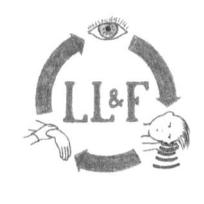

Look—What was the mechanism of injury (MOI)? Can they move their extremities?

Listen—Are they complaining of any neck or back pain?

Feel—Do they have normal sensation in their extremities?

- Upon arrival at the patient's side, you place a hand on the forehead to hold their head still, or you ask someone else to stabilize the cervical spine while you continue the PAS.
- If they are unconscious, or if the mechanism of injury (MOI) indicates possible injury to the spine, continue to immobilize their neck and back.
- Later after completion of the PAS, you will come back and re-examine the spine to see if you can clear it or if you need to continue immobilization of the spine.

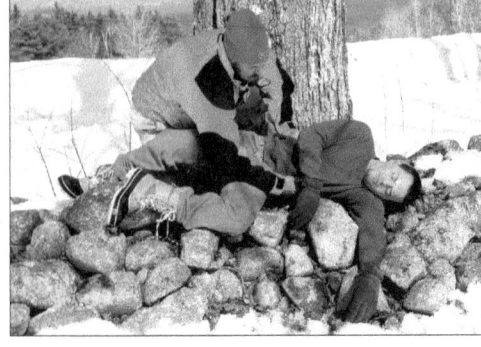

Perform a "chunk check" to check for bleeding.

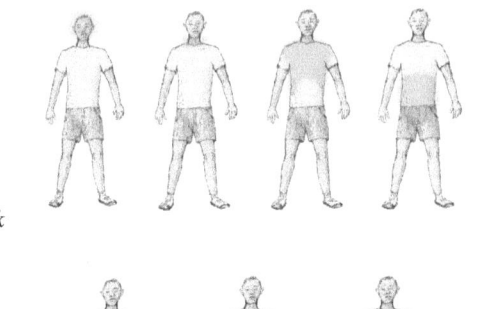

Chunk Check

Environment—Can they stay where they are?

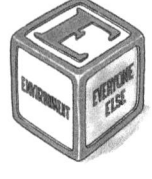
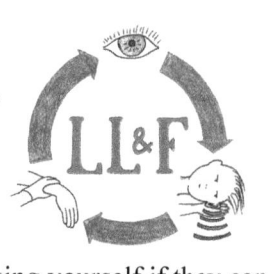
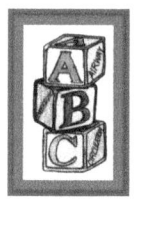

Look—Where are they lying?

Listen—Are they complaining about being hot, cold, or wet?

Feel—Is their skin warm, dry, cold, or wet?

- Right from the moment you arrive at the patient's side, you have to be asking yourself if they can stay where they are or if they need to be moved.
- Whenever possible, you try to keep them lying still until you can complete the PAS and you have a good idea what the injuries are.
- However, this is not always possible, and you may have to move them without knowing the extent of the injuries.
- If a move is necessary, you have to figure out where they can be safely relocated.
- At a minimum and as soon as possible, get them onto an ensolite pad or other soft, insulating material to protect them from the ground.
- If necessary, surround them with warm insulation or provide shade.
- Eventually they will have to be moved into a shelter to protect them from the weather.

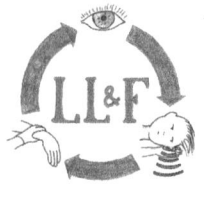

Everyone Else—How is everyone else in the group doing?

Look—How does the rest of the group look?

Listen—Is anyone complaining of being cold, wet, hungry, or thirsty?

Feel—What is the emotional status of the group?

- STOP and consider the whole group.
- How is everyone else doing?
- Is everyone warm and dry and protected from the environment?
- Keep everyone busy.

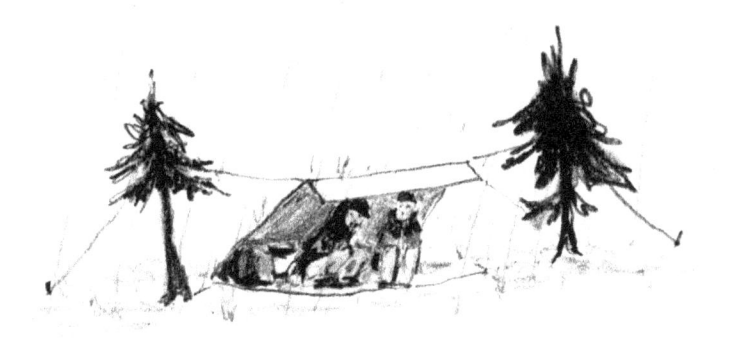

THIRD: STOP—The SECONDARY SURVEY—History of Present Illness, Vital Signs, Patient Exam, AMPLE History, SOAPnote

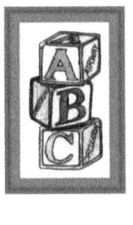

- What happened?—History of Present Illness
- How well are they?—Vital Signs
- What are their injuries?—Patient Exam
- What is their past medical history?—AMPLE History
- What is our patient care plan?—SOAPnote

Upon completion of the Scene Survey and the Primary Survey, the life-threatening problems have been eliminated or managed. Now you have the luxury of time to move on to the Secondary Survey and answer the question, "How hurt are they?" By taking a set of vital signs, performing a patient exam, and taking an AMPLE history, you will be able to determine the extent and severity of the injuries or illness.

History of Present Illness:

- Onset of injury or illness
- Location of pain or injury
- Quality of pain
- Quantity of pain (0 = no pain; 10 = worst pain ever)

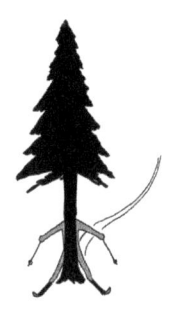

Vital Signs

A person's ability to acquire and utilize oxygen (O_2) is the most important thing. The first responsibility is to make sure the person has an open airway, is breathing, has a pulse, and is not bleeding. Once that is established, you measure and monitor the VITAL SIGNS of the body's major systems in order to determine if a person is getting better, staying the same, or getting worse as a result of injuries, illness, or care provid

A person can live:
- Weeks without food.
- Days without water.
- Hours in a harsh environment without shelter.
- But only SIX MINUTES without oxygen.

What vital signs tell you:
- How well your patient is doing in response to the injury.
- And how serious the injury is.

What vital signs don't tell you:
- What the specific injury is.

Vital signs set the pace:
- Take a set of vital signs every 5–15 minutes.
- They give you a picture over time of how well your patient is doing.
- They give you confidence that you are doing your job and your patient is doing well.

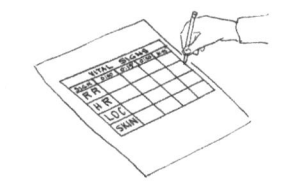

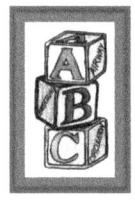

Vital Signs: By System

Respiratory System (airway and lungs)
The oxygen exchange system: "In with the good air and out with the bad."

- Respiratory Rate: Count the number of breaths per minute—normal: 10-30/minute
- Respiratory Effort: Observe; watch them breathe—normal: no effort
- How hard are they working to breathe?
- Ask them if they feel short of breath, or if they are having a hard time breathing.

Circulatory System (heart, blood vessels, and blood)
Transports the oxygen to every cell in the body: "Do not be still, my beating heart."

- Heart Rate: Find the pulse at the wrist and count it for a minute—normal: 50-100 beats/minute
- Effort: May use a blood pressure (bp) cuff or simply check for pulses—normal: all pulses intact
  - If you get a pulse at the wrist, there is a minimum BP of 90mmHg, enough to perfuse the entire body.
  - If you get a pulse at the femoral artery, there is a minimum BP of 70mmHg, enough to perfuse the vital organs and brain.
  - If you get a pulse at the carotid artery, there is a minimum BP of 60mmHg, enough to perfuse only the brain.

Central Nervous System (brain and spinal cord)
Uses oxygen to survive and thrive and establishes the Level of Consciousness (LOC).

- Monitor LOC with the AVPU scale—normal: awake, alert, oriented x 3

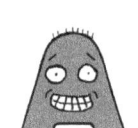

Awake: conscious: how alert are they? —"The lights are on, but is anyone home?"

- Alert and Oriented times one (x1): **person**—they only know who they are (A&O x 1 = bad).
- Alert and Oriented x 2: **place**—they know who they are and where they are (A&O x 2 = better).
- Alert and Oriented x 3: **time**—they know who they are, where they are, the day, week, & year (A&O x 3 = best).

Verbal: unconscious: but do they respond to sound?— "Hello, anyone in there?"

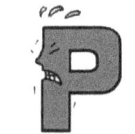

- Speak to them; do they react to hearing their name (attempting to speak, making movement)?
- Do they follow simple commands (blinking, moving a limb)?

Painful: unconscious: but do they respond to pain?—"That's got to hurt."

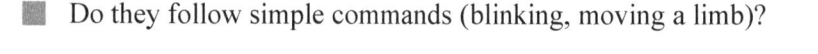

- Does a knuckle rubbed on their sternum elicit a response (guarding, groaning)?
- Is it an appropriate response to pain?

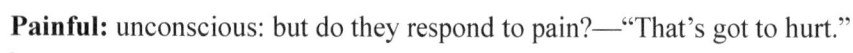

Unresponsive: unconscious, comatose.

- "No one's home."
- No response to verbal or painful stimuli.

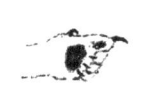

Integumentary System (skin):

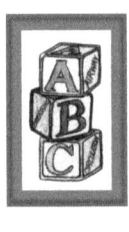

The largest organ in the human body, responsible for thermoregulation. If there is limited oxygen, the brain will prioritize and vasoconstrict the peripheral circulation in the skin, shunting the blood away from the skin to vital organs.

Skin color: varies by individual and race.
- Is there perfusion of blood to the skin?
- Check capillary refill.
- Look at the nonpigmented areas of the body: the nail beds, under the eyelids, in the mouth.

Skin temperature and moisture: not too hot, not too cold.
- Touch their skin on the abdomen and in the axilla (armpit).
- Are they hot or cold to the touch? Are they dry, wet, or sweaty?

HEALTHY SET OF VITAL SIGNS				
Vital Sign	**Time (0:00)**	**Time (0:15)**	**Time (0:30)**	**Time (0:45)**
RR & Effort	16—no effort	12—no effort	12—no effort	12—no effort
HR & Effort (BP by palp)	80 + radial pulse	72 + radial pulse	60 + radial pulse	60 + radial pulse
LOC	A&O x 3	A&O x 3	A&O x 3	A&O x 3
Skin	warm & moist	warm & moist	warm & moist	warm & moist

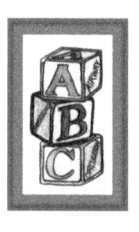

You are going to record what you find using a format called a SOAP note.

S is for "subjective" information (what the patient tells you)

O is for "objective" information (what you observe or find)

A is for your assessment of what is wrong with the patient, or what you suspect is wrong.

P is for your plan to deal with what is wrong.

More on SOAP notes later on...

Vital signs are listed under "O" for objective findings.

The key here is to remember that one set of vital signs does not tell you anything. Vital signs taken at intervals over time tell you if the patients condition is improving, getting worse, or is stable.

An example of what a SOAP note might look like.

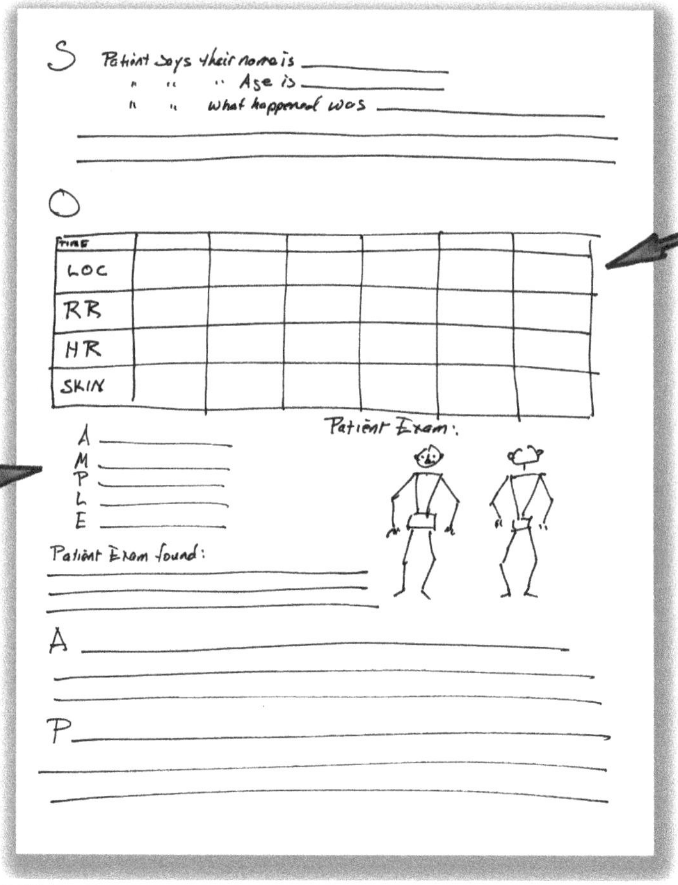

Vital signs go here under "Objective" information.

We will cover AMPLE and assessment later, what is important here is getting an accurate set of vital signs.

Patient Exam—The principles of a thorough search for trouble

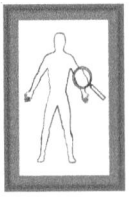

- Hands-on, head-to-toe exam that locates the injuries.
- Done in much the same way as a good massage.
- One person does the entire exam.
- Start at the head; then do: neck—chest—abdomen—legs—arms—back.
- Talk with the patient; explain what you are doing.
- If they complain of pain, ask where it hurts.
- Avoid unnecessary movement.
- History of Present Illness—get a thorough history of what happened.

Principles of the Patient Exam—you are trying to discover all possible injuries by:

INSPECTION: Look for bleeding & wounds, impaled objects, deformities.

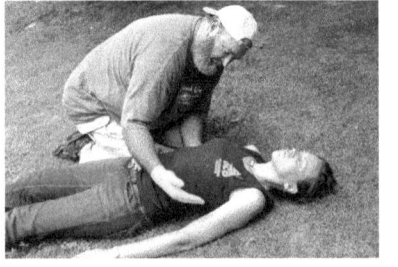

CIRCULATION: Check all four extremities for pulses.

C

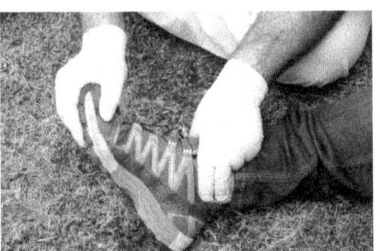

COMPARISON: Check symmetry of body parts.

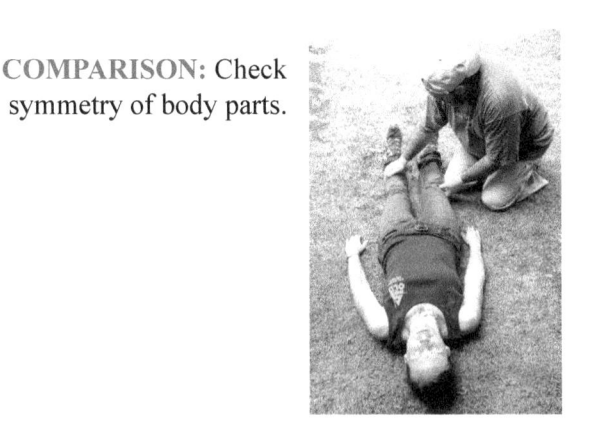

SENSATION: Check all four extremities for sensation.

S

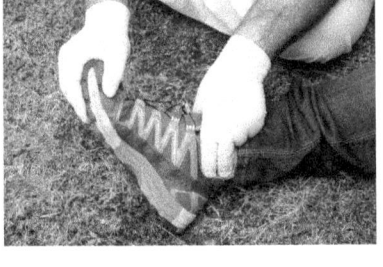

PALPATION: Is there tenderness in muscles, bones, or joints?

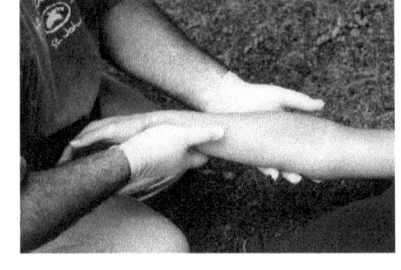

MOTION: Check all four extremities for the ability to move.

M

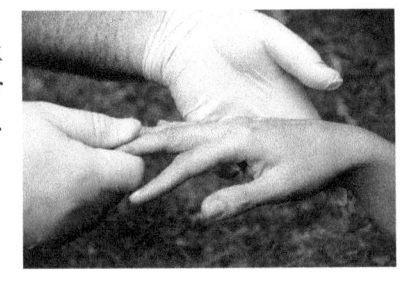

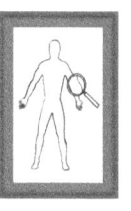

HEAD: Inspect scalp, face, eyes, nose, mouth, ears.

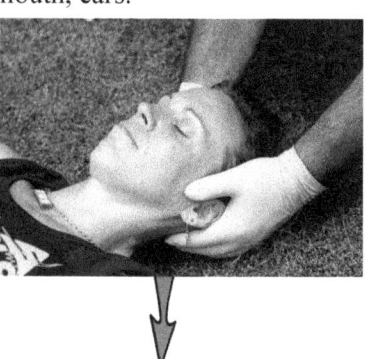

NECK: Palpate cervical spine, inspect trachea.

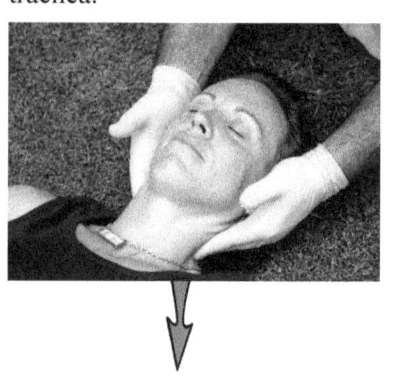

CHEST: Palpate clavicles, shoulder, and compress the rib cage.

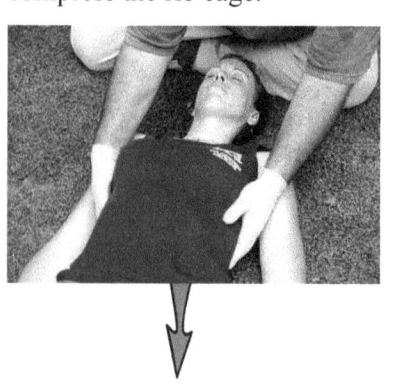

ABDOMEN: Compress the abdomen in the center.

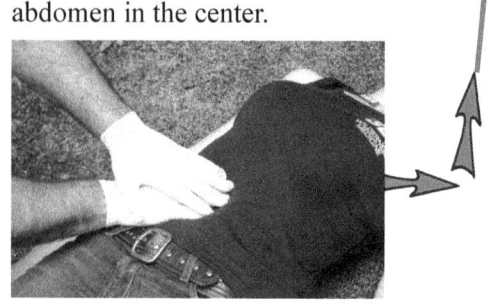

PELVIS: Compress the pelvis front to back and laterally.

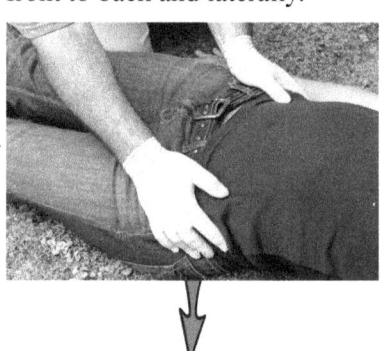

LEGS: Palpate the muscles and ask patient to flex the joints.

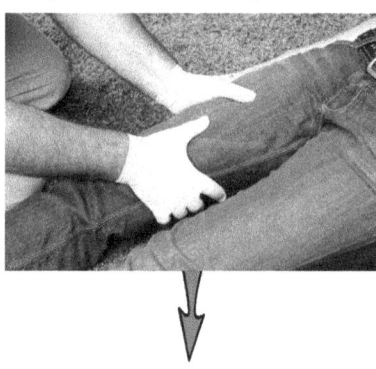

ARMS: Palpate the muscles and ask patient to flex their joints.

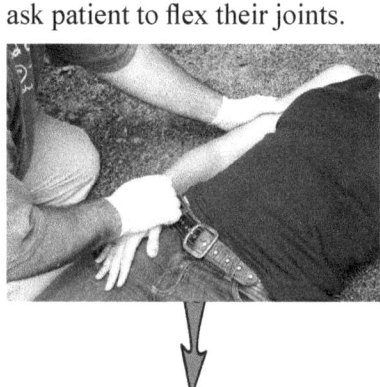

BACK: Palpate the length of the back.

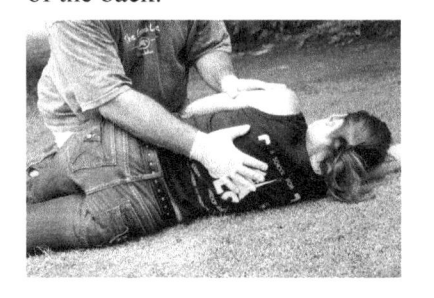

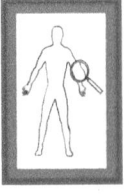

AMPLE History

Everyone has a past medical history that others may not be aware of. This medical history can be very important and can be a factor in providing proper medical care. Use the simple mnemonic of AMPLE to remind yourself of the appropriate questions to ask your patients about their medical history.

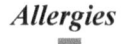

Allergies

- To medications, foods, insects, etc.
- What happens and how is it treated?

Medications

- What medications are they taking (both prescription and over-the-counter)?
- Have they taken their meds today? How often and how much?

Previous Injury or Illness

- Any recent or past injury or illness that could contribute to the current problem?

Last Input and Output

- When was the last time they ate or drank?
- What did they eat and drink?
- When was the last time they voided or had a bowel movement?

Events leading up to the crisis

- What led up to or occurred just prior to the critical event?

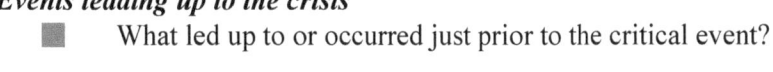

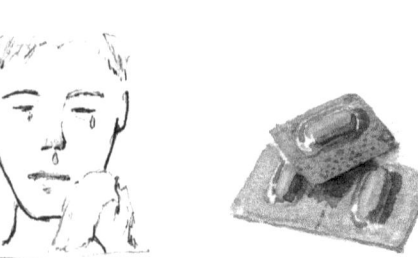

Allergies?   *Medications?*   *History?*   *Last in, last out*

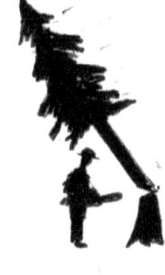

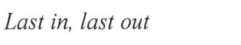

What happened.

SOAPnote

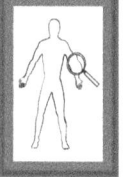

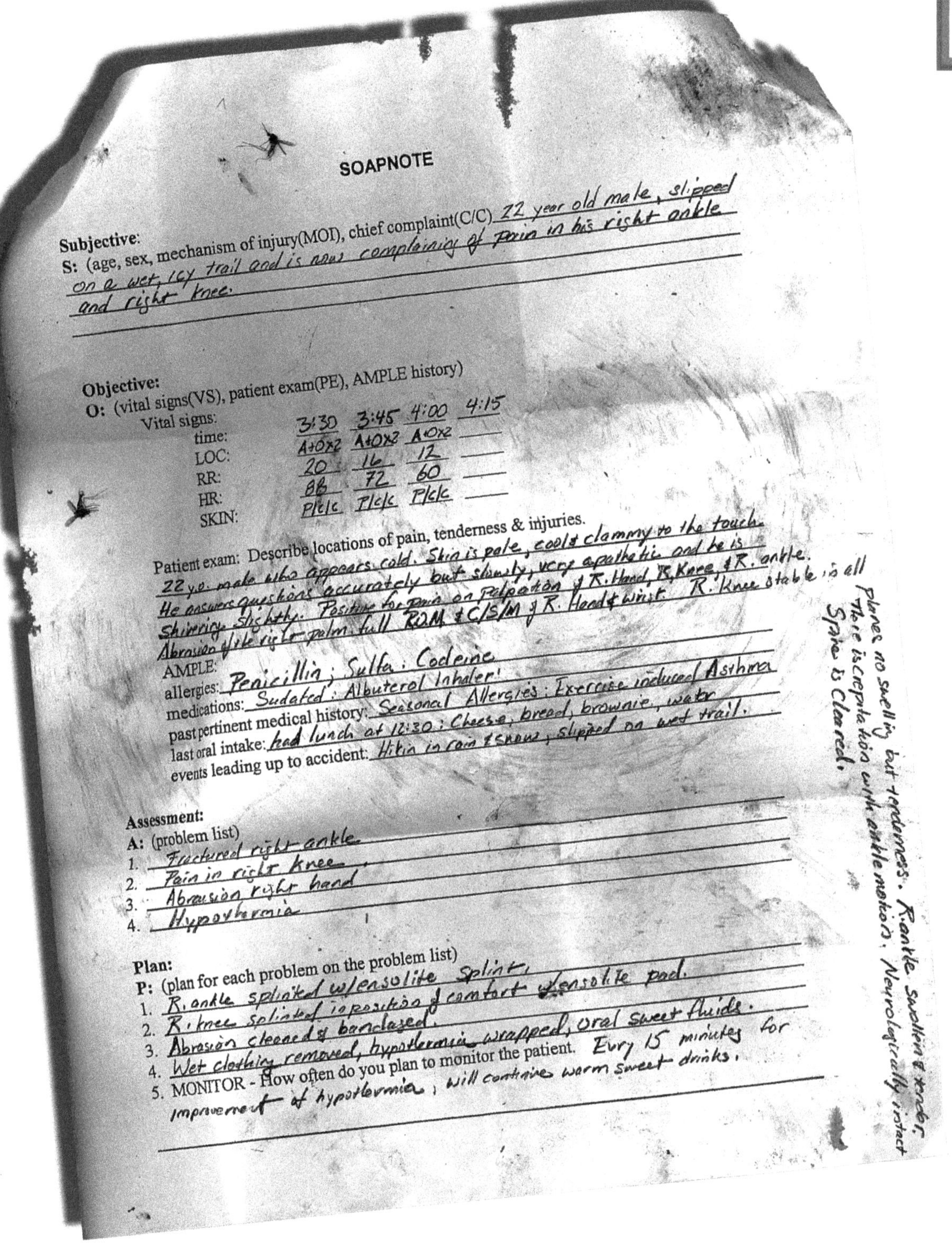

SOAPNOTE

Subjective:
S: (age, sex, mechanism of injury(MOI), chief complaint(C/C) _22 year old male, slipped_
on a wet, icy trail and is now complaining of Pain in his right ankle
and right knee.

Objective:
O: (vital signs(VS), patient exam(PE), AMPLE history)

Vital signs:

time:	3:30	3:45	4:00	4:15
LOC:	A+O×2	A+O×3	A+O×2	
RR:	20	16	12	
HR:	88	72	60	
SKIN:	P/c/c	P/c/c	P/c/c	

Patient exam: Describe locations of pain, tenderness & injuries.
22 y.o. male who appears cold. Skin is pale, cool & clammy to the touch.
He answers questions accurately but slowly, very apathetic and he is
Shivering slightly. Positive for Pain on Palpation of R. Hand, R. Knee & R. ankle.
Abrasion of the right palm. full ROM & C/S/M of R. Hand & Wrist. R. Knee & table is all

AMPLE:
allergies: _Penicillin, Sulfa, Codeine_
medications: _Sudafed, Albuterol Inhaler_
past pertinent medical history: _Seasonal Allergies, Exercise induced Asthma_
last oral intake: _had lunch at 12:30, Cheese, bread, brownie, water_
events leading up to accident: _Hikin in rain & snow, slipped on wet trail._

Assessment:
A: (problem list)
1. _Fractured right ankle_
2. _Pain in right knee_
3. _Abrasion right hand_
4. _Hypothermia_

Plan:
P: (plan for each problem on the problem list)
1. _R. ankle splinted w/ensolite splint._
2. _R. knee splinted in position of comfort of ensolite pad._
3. _Abrasion cleaned & bandaged._
4. _Wet clothing removed, hypothermia wrapped, oral sweet fluids._
5. MONITOR - How often do you plan to monitor the patient. _Evry 15 minutes for_
improvement of hypothermia, will continue warm sweet drinks.

planes no swelling but tenderness. R. ankle swelling & tender
There is crepitation with ankle motion. Neurologically intact
Spine is Cleared.

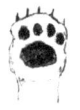

PATIENT ASSESSMENT CHECK LIST

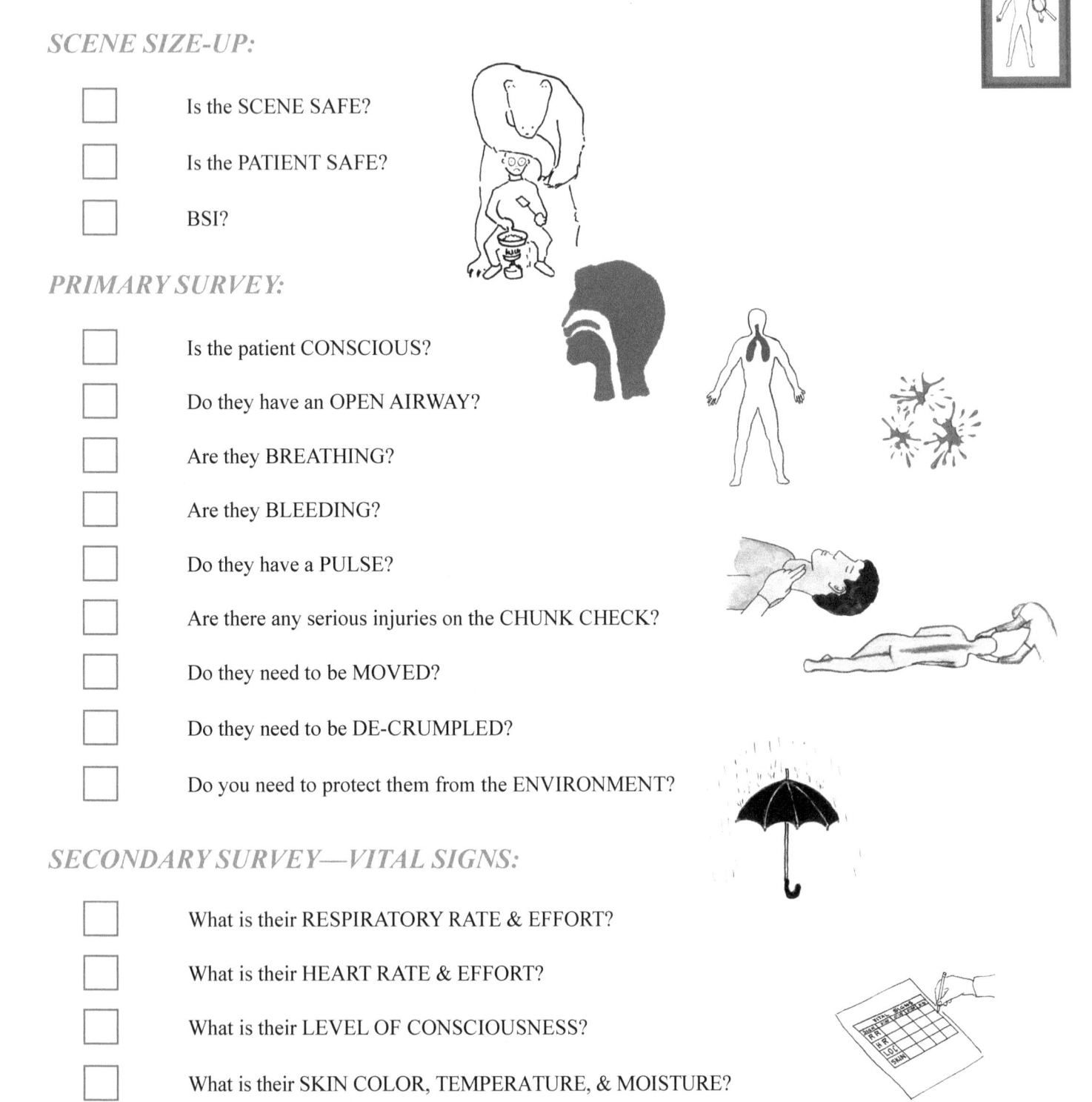

SCENE SIZE-UP:

☐ Is the SCENE SAFE?

☐ Is the PATIENT SAFE?

☐ BSI?

PRIMARY SURVEY:

☐ Is the patient CONSCIOUS?

☐ Do they have an OPEN AIRWAY?

☐ Are they BREATHING?

☐ Are they BLEEDING?

☐ Do they have a PULSE?

☐ Are there any serious injuries on the CHUNK CHECK?

☐ Do they need to be MOVED?

☐ Do they need to be DE-CRUMPLED?

☐ Do you need to protect them from the ENVIRONMENT?

SECONDARY SURVEY—VITAL SIGNS:

☐ What is their RESPIRATORY RATE & EFFORT?

☐ What is their HEART RATE & EFFORT?

☐ What is their LEVEL OF CONSCIOUSNESS?

☐ What is their SKIN COLOR, TEMPERATURE, & MOISTURE?

SECONDARY SURVEY—PATIENT EXAM:

☐   HEAD—scalp, face, eyes, nose, mouth

☐   NECK—spine, trachea

☐   CHEST—clavicles, shoulders, ribs

☐   ABDOMEN—compress the abdomen

☐   PELVIS—compress the pelvis, anterior/posterior and lateral

☐   LEGS—circulation, sensation, and motion

☐   ARMS—circulation, sensation, and motion

☐   BACK—log roll and palpate the length of the spine

SECONDARY SURVEY—AMPLE HISTORY:

☐   ALLERGY—allergy to drugs, foods, insects, etc.

☐   MEDS—prescription and non-prescription drugs

☐   PREVIOUS—significant past medical history, surgeries, etc.

☐   LAST—last intake & last output

☐   EVENT—events leading up to this crisis

SOAPNOTE—RECORD VITAL INFORMATION:
ON-GOING ASSESSMENT

☐   Record patient data.

☐   Re-SOAP every 15 minutes.

FOURTH: STOP—Rescue Survey—how to get help

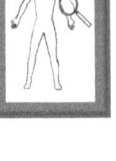

The Patient Assessment System has been completed. You now combine the patient's condition with the group's condition and determine if you need help from rescuers.

Patient's condition:
- Continuously monitor the patient's condition.
- Re-SOAP every 15 minutes.

    S: are they hungry, thirsty, in pain, need to go to the bathroom?

    O: take and record a complete set of vital signs, check all splints and bandages for circulation.

    A: is assessment the same?

    P: is the plan the same?

Group's condition:
- How well is each individual in the group doing: hungry, thirsty, anxious?
- How well-prepared is the group to stay put and bivouac?

Decisions:
- Do you need to evacuate the patient or can you all go on?
- If evacuation is needed, send for help.
- While waiting for rescue—build a bivouac.

Sending for help:
- Send two to get help if possible.
- Send out a SOAPnote on the patient.
- Send out a list of the remaining group and how well-prepared they are to bivouac.
- Send out a map with your exact location and time marked on it.

While waiting for help to arrive:
- Keep spirits up, be positive, reassure, make sure everyone has something to do.
- Create light and warmth; build a fire, keep everyone warm and dry.
- Make yourselves big, easy to find.
- Continuously monitor your patient and the other members of your group.

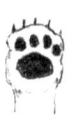

PATIENT LIFTING & MOVING TECHNIQUES

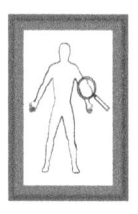

When an injury occurs, it is important to keep the wounded person lying still, as they may not know how seriously they are hurt.

The very first component of patient care you will need to provide is to safely lift or move the patient to another location. This is to protect them from further harm or protect them from the environment. This may occur anytime during the Initial Assessment, Primary Survey, or Secondary Survey.

- ☑ Are they in immediate danger from rock fall, ice fall, avalanche, etc.?

- ☑ Are they lying in water?

- ☑ Are they lying on frozen ground or snow?

- ☑ Are they lying on sharp jagged rocks or other debris?

- ☑ Are they generally in harm's way?

If your patient is in harm's way, you are also in harm's way. One victim is enough.

When possible, try to perform a patient exam or chunk check before moving your patient so you have an idea of what the injuries are.

Personal Safety Precautions:

- ☑ Know your own strength and physical limitations.

- ☑ Work together—get as many hands on the patient as possible; many hands make light work.

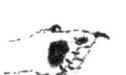

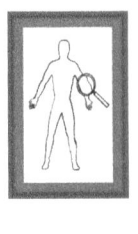

The cardinal rule of moving hurt people...

It is always safe to move someone from the position of injury to the position of function.

...but

Avoid flexion of the head and neck.

- May move the head & neck into neutral position, but do not flex forward.
- Avoid rotation of the pelvis out of alignment with the shoulders.
- May line up the shoulders and the pelvis, but do not rotate out of alignment.

POSITIONS:

SUPINE: Lying flat on your back.

PRONE: Lying flat on your chest & stomach.

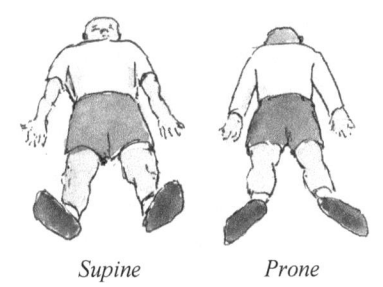

Supine   *Prone*

RECOVERY POSITION: 3/4 prone position used to maintain the airway.

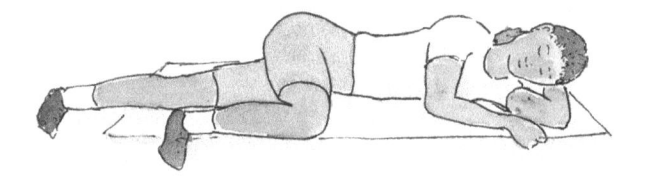

The recovery position.

When lifting, use proper body mechanics:

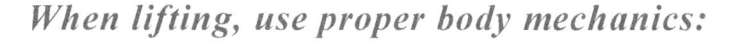

- Lift with your legs.
- Keep your back straight and your butt down.
- Try not to overreach or twist.
- Keep the weight as close to your body as possible.
- Use assists such as blankets, rain flies, or ensolite pads.

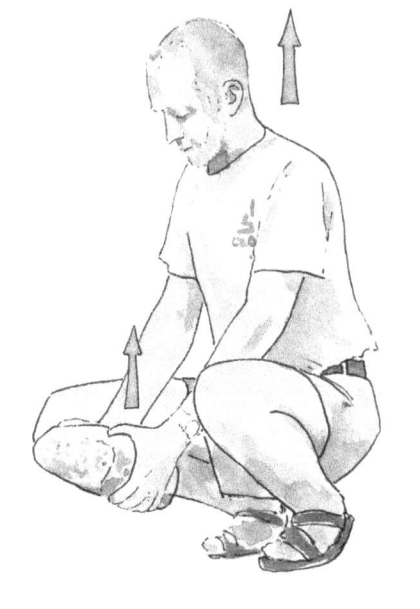

Always lift properly.

LIFTING AND MOVING:

LOG ROLL: Keeping the head, shoulders, and pelvis in line, roll the patient onto their side.

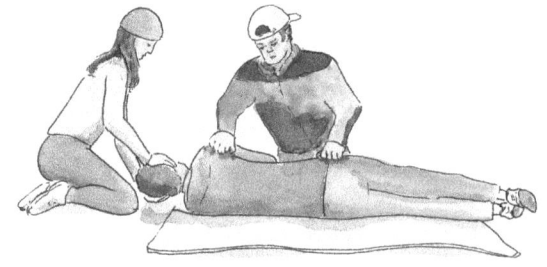
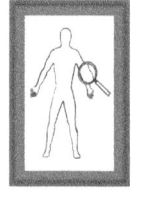

MOVE AS A UNIT: With many hands on, move the person as if they were frozen stiff.

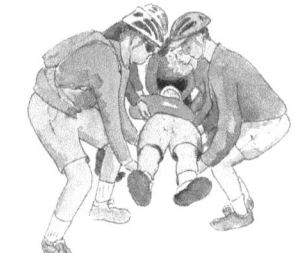

DRAGS: Drag them by their clothing or on a pad.

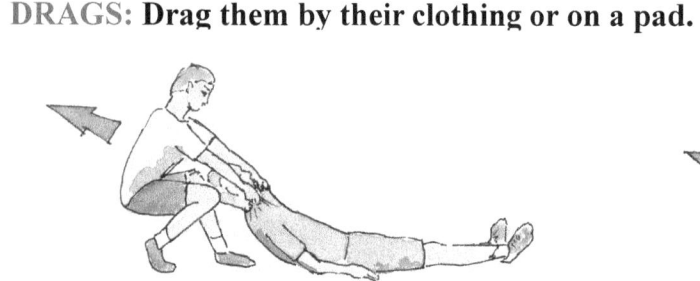

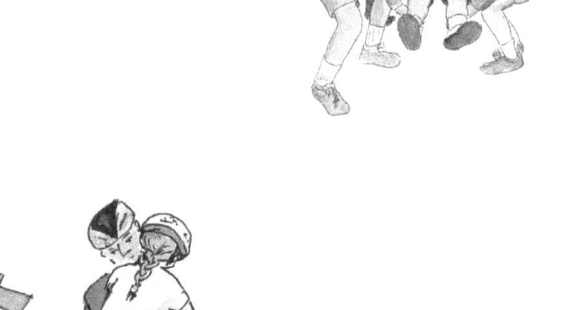

TRANSFERS & CARRIES: With many hands, pick them up and walk:

ONE-PERSON: **Roll onto a pad to drag.**

TWO-PERSON: **May be able to carry or drag.**

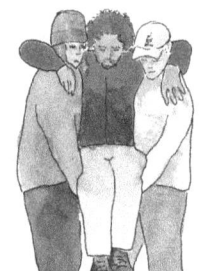
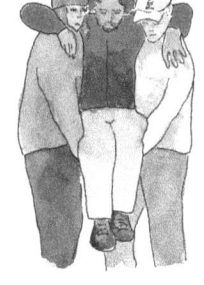

MANY PERSONS: **Much easier, many hands on.**

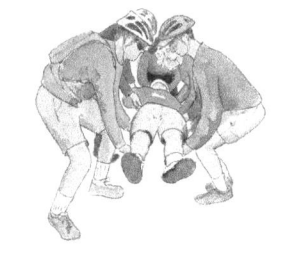

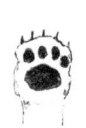

SHOCK

A condition in which the cardiovascular system fails to provide sufficient circulation to every part of the body causing tissues to eventually suffer from a lack of oxygen.

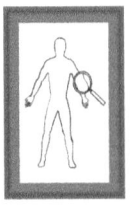

The CARDIOVASCULAR SYSTEM consists of:

- Heart—pumps the blood.
- Blood vessels—carry and distribute the blood.
- Blood—carries the oxygen.

Shock is a compensatory mechanism designed to keep the brain well-oxygenated during times of cardiovascular insufficiency by:

- Vasoconstricting the peripheral circulation, thus pooling blood into the body core,
- Increasing the heart rate, which sends more blood to the brain, and
- Increasing respiratory rate to maximize the amount of oxygen in the blood.

- These COMPENSATORY MECHANISMS occur whenever the BRAIN perceives a threat or crisis, real or not, and puts the cardiovascular system on ALERT STATUS. The ALERT STATUS is transient and self-correcting. SHOCK is the compensatory mechanism caused by failure of the cardiovascular system in its effort to maintain circulation and thus oxygen to the brain.
- In SHOCK the compensatory mechanism prioritizes the blood flow from the heart to the lungs to the brain. The only other organs involved are the liver and kidneys.
- Once injuries are properly treated, the shock condition or Alert Status should cease and the vital signs return to normal. If not, the person is in life-threatening shock.
- Initially shock status is a life-saving condition that preserves blood flow to the brain, but SHOCK KILLS if it continues for too long. You have to find the underlying cause.

Causes of shock:

- HYPOVOLEMIC: **LOW VOLUME** caused by decreased blood volume due to blood loss or dehydration from sweating, diarrhea, vomiting, or a burn.
- CARDIOGENIC: **LOW FLOW** caused by pump failure, i.e. a heart attack.
- NEUROGENIC: **LOW PRESSURE** caused by vasodilation, a loss of vascular tone, that results in increased vascular space. Caused by a spinal cord injury, an acute allergic reaction, or a life-threatening systemic infection, "blood poisoning," or septic shock.

SIGNS & SYMPTOMS

Individuals in shock are not quite "there."

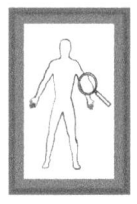

- They are distant.
- They stare off into space or may be unconscious.
- They may not know you are there.
- They may not feel pain or respond to pain.
- They may have an obvious wound or injury that they ignore.
- They may try to walk on a broken leg or use a broken arm.
- They do not know how seriously they are injured.
- They may have a sense of impending doom.

- LOC: restless, anxious, may be disoriented,
- RR: rapid & shallow (increased respiratory rate, more oxygen),
- HR: rapid & weak & thready (increased heart rate, to deliver more blood to the brain),
- SKIN: pale, cool, clammy (due to the vasoconstriction of the capillaries in the skin),
- May collapse; typically nauseous and may vomit.

CARE & TREATMENT:

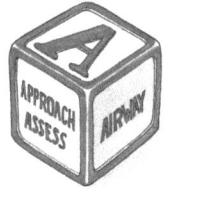

- ☑ AIRWAY, AIRWAY, AIRWAY.
- ☑ Control BLEEDING to minimize blood loss.
- ☑ FIND AND TREAT THE UNDERLYING CAUSE.
- ☑ Treat all injuries to minimize pain.
- ☑ Keep them lying flat in a position of comfort; may elevate the legs.
- ☑ Protect from the environment; maintain body temperature.
- ☑ Monitor vital signs, reassure, & get help.

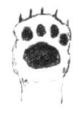

Vital Sign	Time (			
RR & Effort	16—no ef			
HR & Effort (BP by palp)	80 + radial pulse	72 + radial pulse	60 + radial pulse	60 + radial pulse
LOC	A&O x 3	A&O x 3	A&O x 3	A&O x 3
Skin	warm & moist	warm & moist	warm & moist	warm & moist

VITAL SIGNS IN SHOCK				
Vital Sign	Time (0:00)	Time (0:15)	Time (0:30)	Time (0:45)
RR & Effort	16—no effort	12—no effort	20—no effort	30—with effort
HR & Effort (BP by palp)	80 + radial pulse	72 + radial pulse	80 + radial pulse	100 + carotid pulse
LOC	A&O x 3	A&O x 3	A&O x 3 + anxious	A&O x 2 + anxious
Skin	warm & moist	warm & moist	pale & cool	pale, cool, & clammy

Children and Shock:

A child's reaction to shock is different than an adult, in that they are able to compensate extremely well by vasoconstricting the peripheral circulation in the skin. Therefore, one of the first signs of compensatory shock in a child is vasoconstriction of the vasculature in the skin resulting in a delayed capillary refill, pallor, and coolness of the skin. When this occurs in a child look for and treat the underlying cause of shock.

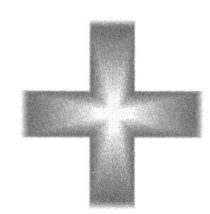

CHAPTER TWO

TRAUMA: MUSCULOSKELETAL INJURIES
Strains, Sprains, and Fractures

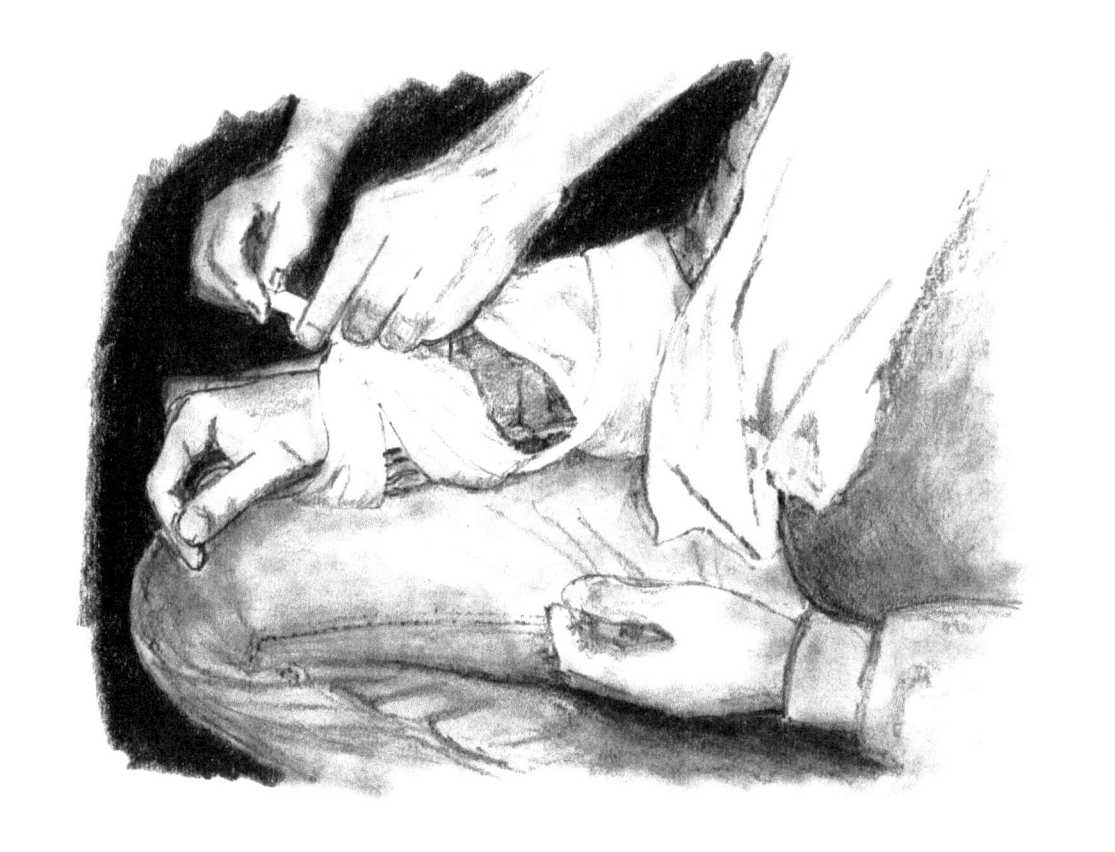

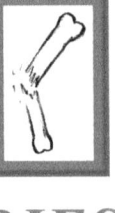

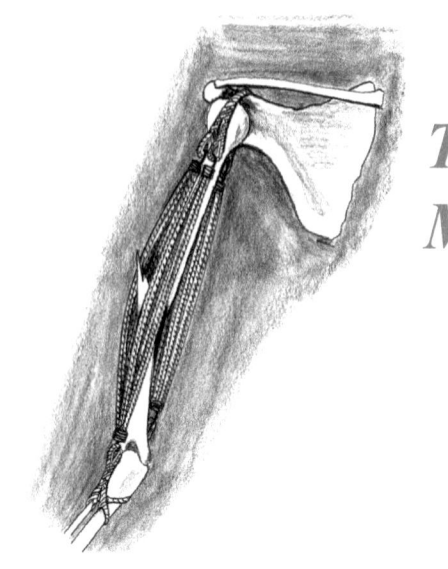

TRAUMA: MUSCULOSKELETAL INJURIES

MUSCULOSKELETAL SYSTEM (BONES, MUSCLES, TENDONS, LIGAMENTS)

When your musculoskeletal system is working properly, this framework of bones, muscles, tendons, ligaments, and cartilage is what holds you up and allows you to move and function.

WHAT THEY DO:

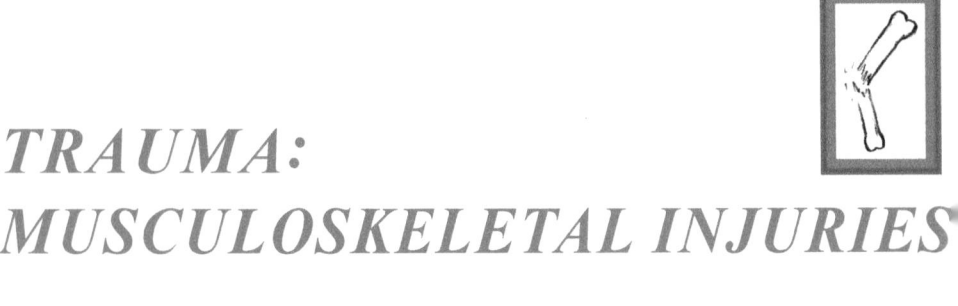

- **BONES** provide the structure to which everything attaches. Bones also store calcium and produce blood cells in the bone marrow.

- **CARTILAGE** acts as a lubricated pad between bones so that your joints can flex or rotate smoothly. Cartilage also provides support for muscle in areas where more flexibility than bone is needed (like your ears).

- **SYNOVIAL FLUID** is the lubricant in the joint space and is produced by the synovial lining of the joint capsule.

- **MUSCLES** are like bundles of bungee cords. They contract or relax in response to signals sent from your brain through your central nervous system, which flexes your joints and allows you to move. Muscles also provide some padding and protection for nerve-bundles, arteries, and veins.

- **LIGAMENTS** are like nylon cords and attach bones to other bones. They maintain proper range of motion.

- **TENDONS** are ties connecting muscle to bone. They span joints and allow for movement.

MUSCULOSKELETAL SYSTEM FUNCTIONS:

- Movement.
- Protection of underlying structures.
- Calcium storage.
- Blood cell production (Hematopoiesis).
- Heat production.
- Cosmesis (your muscles and bones determine how you look).

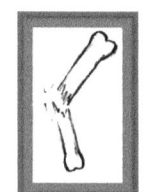

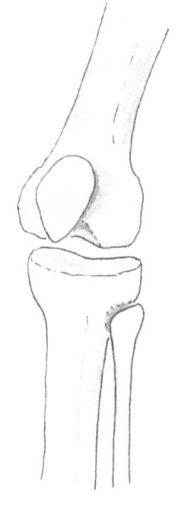 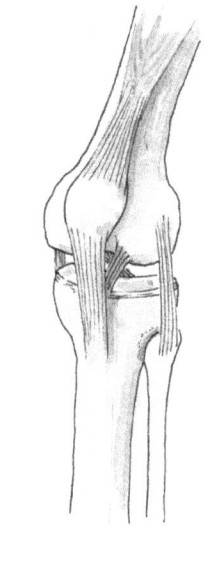 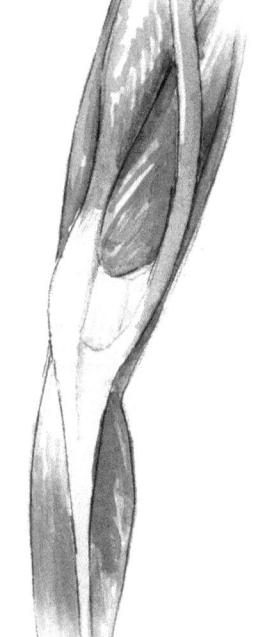 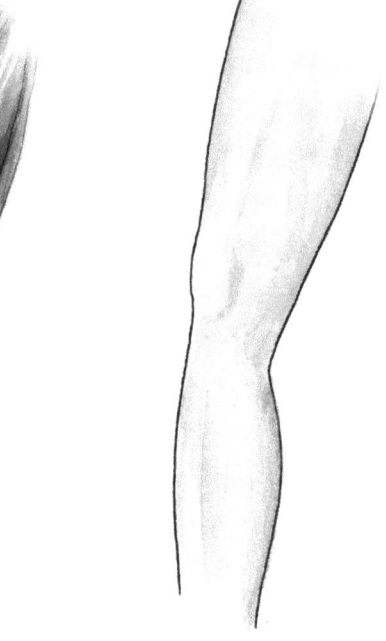

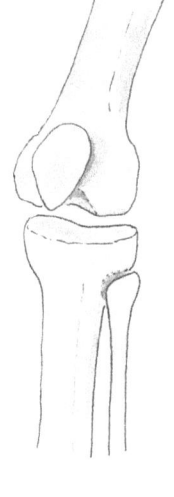

distal

proximal

ANATOMICAL POSITION

When describing the position of parts of the body in relationship to each other, parts that are farther away from the core of the body are described as "DISTAL" and parts that are closer to the core of the body are "PROXIMAL."

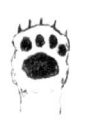

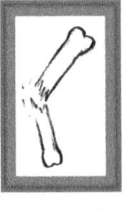

TYPES OF MUSCULOSKELETAL INJURIES:

- ■ Sprains and Strains—twisting and pulling damage to the supporting structure of joints (ligaments, muscles, and tendons) are by far the most common backcountry injuries.
- ■ Fractures—breaks of the hard outer layer of bone can be particularly dangerous because the sharp ends of the bones can cause damage to the surrounding muscle, nerves, and blood vessels.

SPRAINS & STRAINS:

Signs and Symptoms:

☑ Generalized pain around a joint, no point tenderness.

☑ Pain with movement of the joint.

☑ Minimal pain with weight-bearing.

☑ Swelling can be dramatic.

☑ May become discolored over time, "black and blue" (ecchymosis).

Treatment: the primary goal is to minimize swelling by using RICE:

☑ Rest: stop and sit down; this slows circulation.

☑ Ice: causes vasoconstriction, decreasing circulation—ice, snow, or wet.

☑ Compression: decreases circulation and room for swelling; the less it swells the faster it will heal.

☑ Elevation: decreases circulation.

☑ Immobilize & support the affected joint.

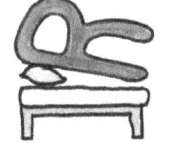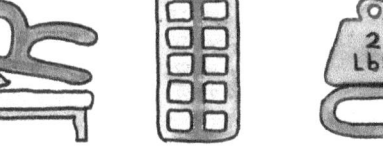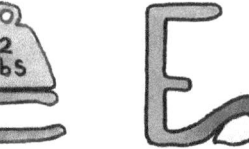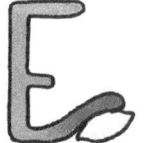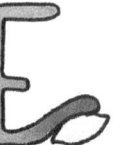

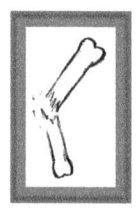

FRACTURES:

- Bones are made up of a hard outer layer of compact bone and an inner soft area of bone marrow.
- A fracture occurs when enough force is exerted against a bone to break the outer compact bone.

EVALUATING A MUSCULOSKELETAL INJURY:

	SPRAIN	*FRACTURE*
Look—What do you see when you examine the injury?		
Do they have normal movement and function?	Usually	No
Are they guarding the injury?	Slightly	Yes
Do you see any deformity or angulations?	No	Yes
Do you see any discoloration or swelling?	Maybe	Yes
Listen—Talk to the patient; what do they say?		
What happened?		
What was the Mechanism Of Injury (MOI)?		
Where does it hurt?		
Did they feel anything snap, crack, or pop?	Maybe	Usually
Feel—What do you feel when you examine the injury?		
Is there good Circulation, Sensation, and Motion (CSM)?	Usually	Maybe
Is there point tenderness?	No	Yes
Is there crepitation (the sound of broken bones grinding)?	No	Yes

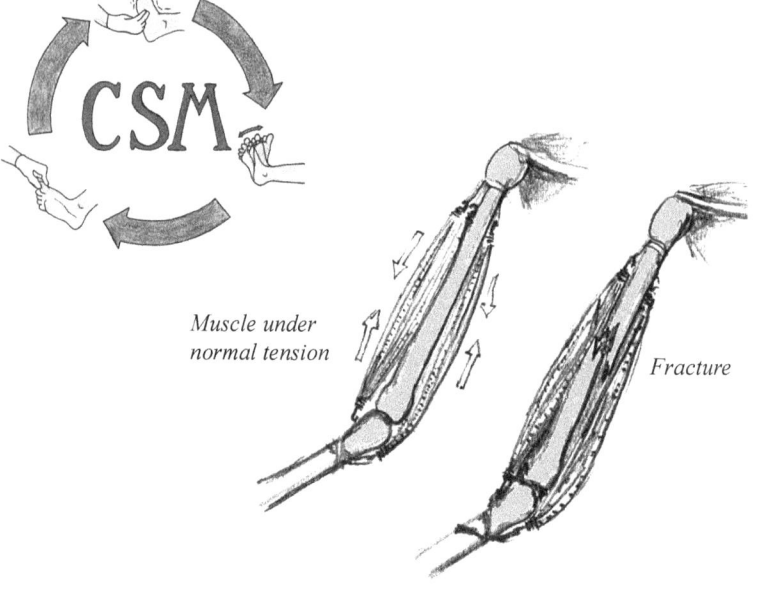

Muscle under normal tension

Fracture

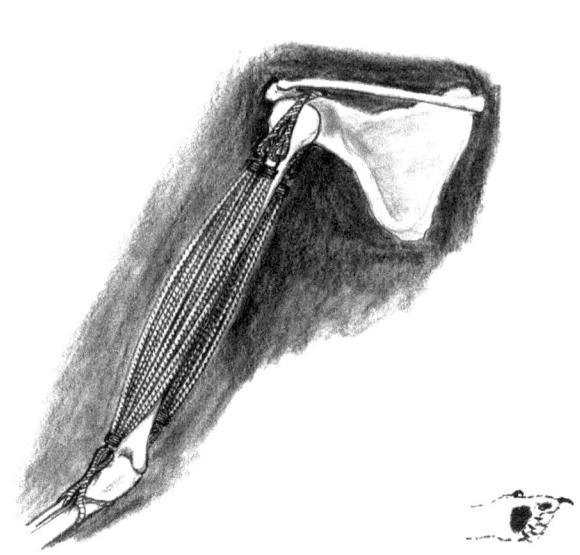

If the Mechanism of Injury indicates a possible fracture, treat as such.

WHEN IN DOUBT, SPLINT!

THE PRINCIPLES OF SPLINTING:

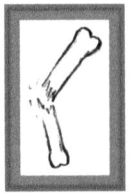

☑ Can the injury be immobilized in the position found? **Check circulation**.

☑ If not, pull **traction-in-line** to slowly and gently move the extremity into proper anatomical alignment. This establishes and maintains circulation distal to the site of the injury.

☑ Create a rigid but **well-padded** splint (well-insulated in winter); fill all voids.

☑ Immobilize the **entire extremity**, including the joint above and below the site of the injury.

☑ **Monitor** all splints; check C/S/M distal to the site of the injury every fifteen minutes.

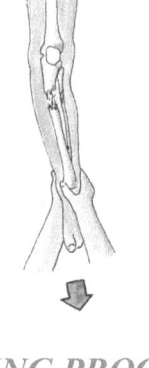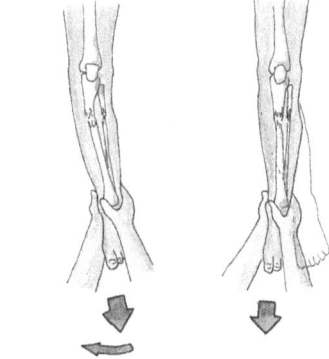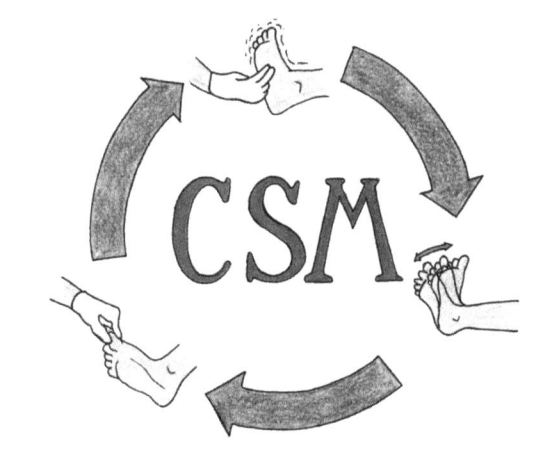

SPLINTING PROCEDURES:

Improvise cervical collar:

- Used to protect neck.
- Soft, conforms to neck.
- Warm.
- Comfortable.

Arm sling & swathe—uses:

- Dislocated shoulder.
- Fractured clavicle.
- Fractured humerus.
- Fractured forearm, wrist, hand.
- Elbow injury.
- Fractured ribs.

Forearm splint:

- Rigid splint with sticks, pack stays, etc. used with arm sling and swathe.

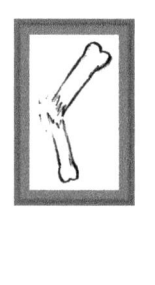

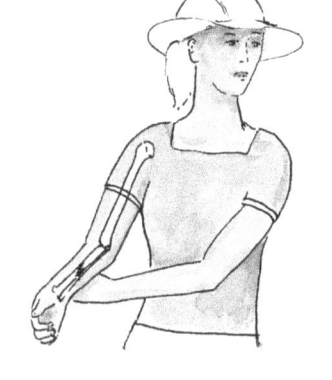
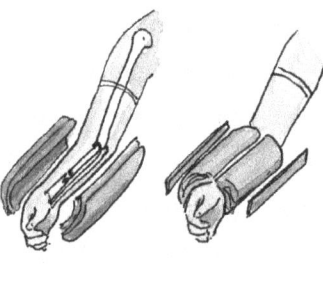
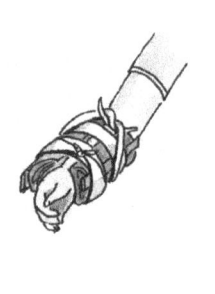
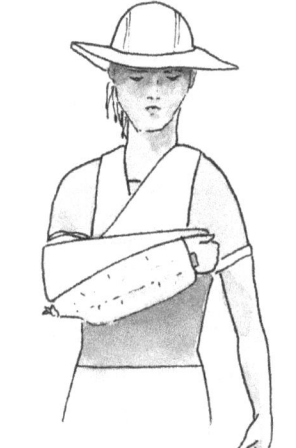

Improvised lower leg & ankle splint:

- Rigid splint with sticks, poles, skis, etc.
- Ensolite pad splint.

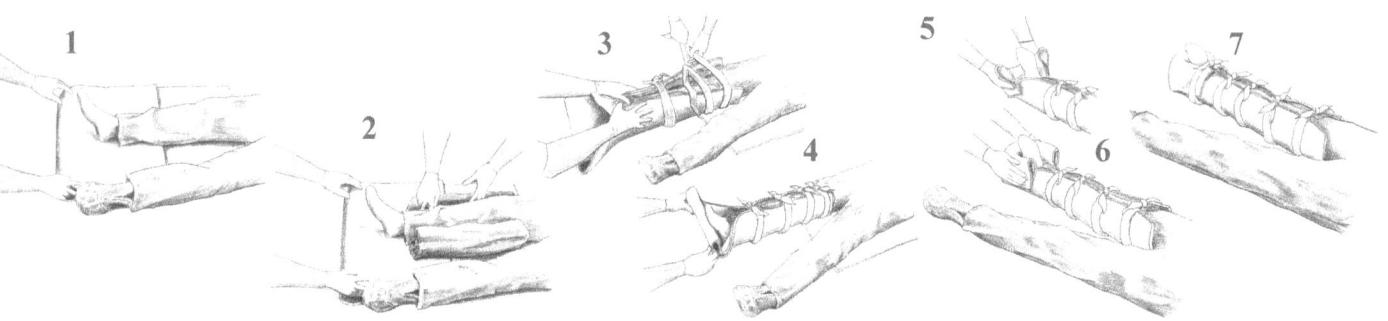

Improvised knee splint:

- Splint knee in position of comfort (30⁰ +/-).
- Place padding in the hollow behind the knee.

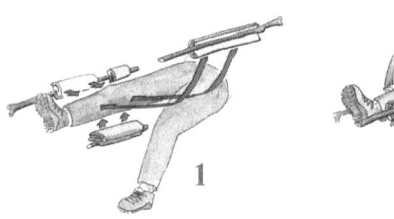
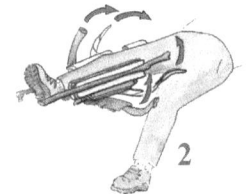
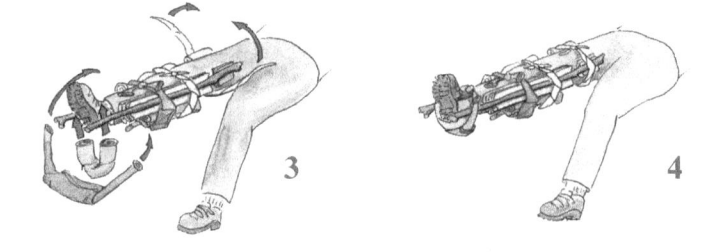

Sprained ankle bandage:

- To splint a fractured ankle or support a sprained ankle.

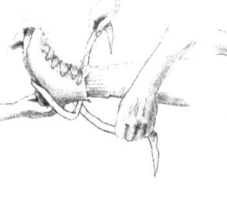
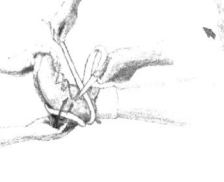
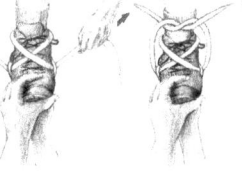
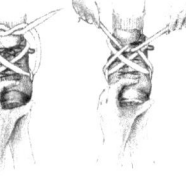
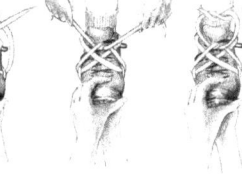
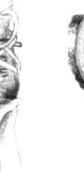
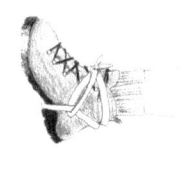
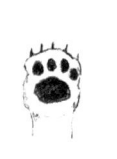
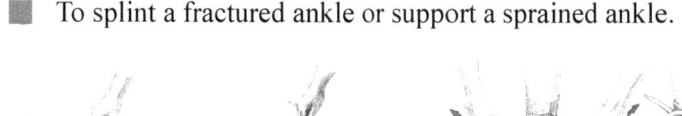

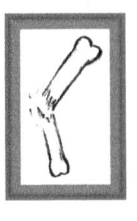

SPINAL CORD INJURY MANAGEMENT:

- ■ Pre-hospital personnel are trained to treat all possible spinal cord injuries based on the Mechanism Of Injury (MOI) as well as symptoms and complaints.

- ■ It is important in the wild environment for rescuers to recognize a possible back injury based on MOI, but it is equally important that they be able to rule it out or "clear the spine" by a proper history and physical exam in order to avoid an unnecessary litter evacuation.

- ■ Spinal assessment—to clear the spine—is not performed until after the patient assessment system has been completed and it is appropriate to evaluate and potentially clear the spine of any possible injury.

Method of clearing the spine: Patient must meet all of these criteria to clear the spine.

- ■ Patient must be sober, conscious, coherent, and oriented x 3, in person, place, & time.

- ■ Patient has no painful distracting injuries (e.g. fractured femur, compound fracture, burn).

- ■ Patient does not complain of any pain the entire length of the back.

- ■ Patient does not have radiating pain, paresthesias (tingling), paralysis, or numbness in any of their extremities.

- ■ Patient has intact sensation and motion in all four extremities unless local injury.

- ■ Patient has no tenderness on physical exam along the entire length of the back.

- ■ Without assistance, the patient is able to flex, extend, and rotate neck, upper, and lower back without pain or discomfort, and this movement is symmetrical without locking sensation or limited range of motion.

- ■ You can always move the patient into proper anatomical position.

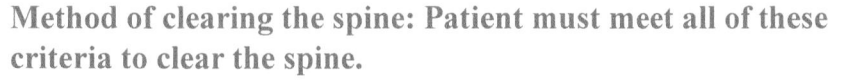

C7

T12

L5

sacrum & coccyx

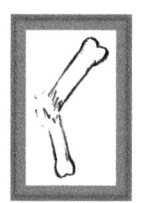

SPINAL CORD INJURY MANAGEMENT:

- It is more important to know how to move an injured person, to protect them from further injury than it is to know how to backboard them.
- Cervical spine is at risk with flexion; do not lift head.
- Lumbar spine is at risk with rotation; keep shoulders, and hips aligned.
- Lifting and moving techniques were discussed with Patient Assessment.

Cervical Collars:

- You can improvise very comfortable and immobilizing soft blanket and horseshoe collars out of materials such as a pile jacket, blanket, or ensolite pad. They provide support, comfort, and warmth.

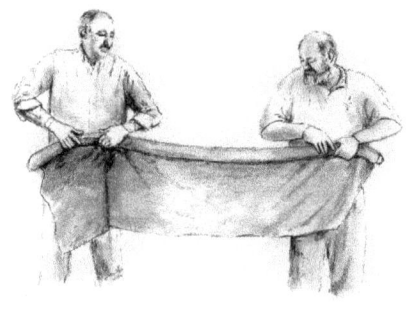
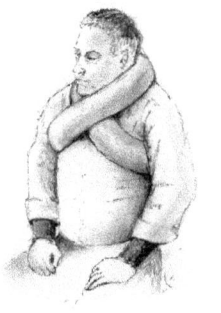

Backboards:

- Backboards or litters are only used by rescue teams for transport.
- While waiting for help to arrive, simply keep the patient still, comfortable, and warm.
- Protect them from the cold or hot ground.
- Remember not to flex the neck! Keep the spine straight by log rolling the patient.

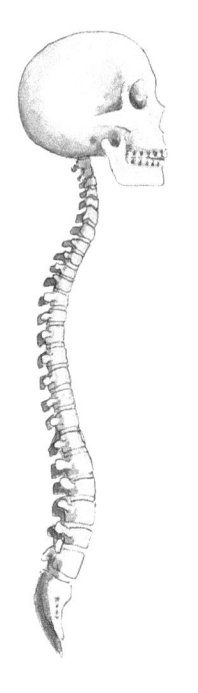
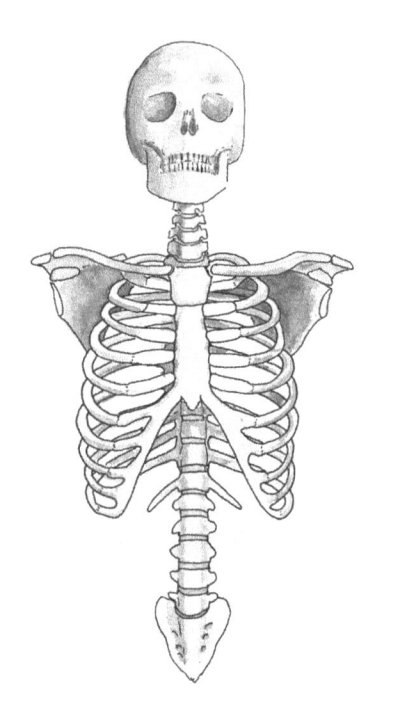

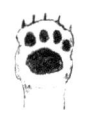

41

— NOTES —

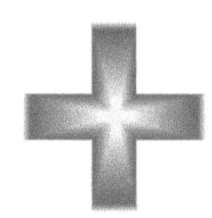

CHAPTER THREE

ENVIRONMENTAL EMERGENCIES & SURVIVAL SKILLS
How To Survive and Thrive in the World

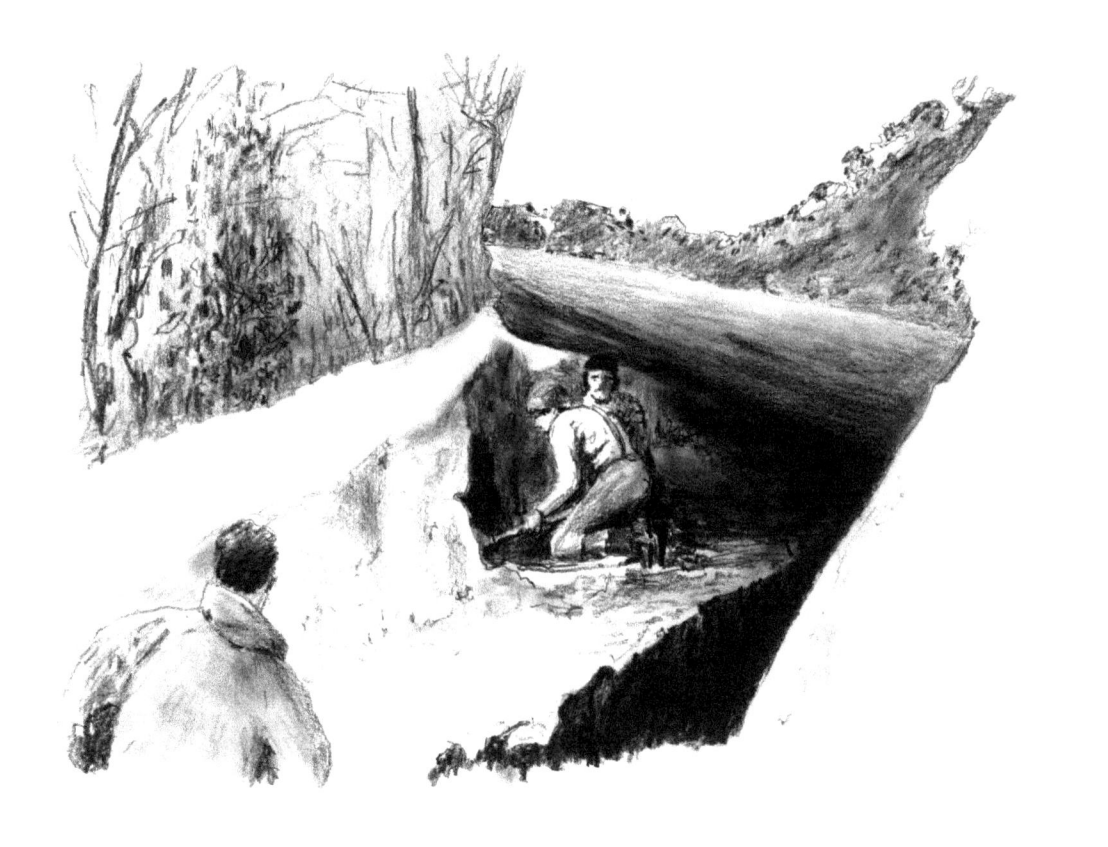

ENVIRONMENTAL EMERGENCIES AND SURVIVAL SKILLS:

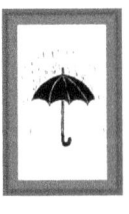

What are your biggest risks from the environment?

On Average:

3500 people die from drowning each year in the U.S.*

700 to 1300 die from cold

600 die from heat related injuries

48.5 die from bee/hornet/wasp stings

48 die from lightning strikes

6.6 die from spider bites

5.2 die from snakebite

1 to 3 die from rabies

2 die as a result of bear attack

However, percentage wise, your greatest risk in the U.S. might be from ticks since 59,262 people got sick from tick-born diseases in 2017.

Before you examine environmental threats, it is critical that you understand how your body reacts to changes in your environment. You have characteristics that make you both wonderfully suited to your environment and yet terribly susceptible to its fluctuations.

THE HUMAN ANIMAL

- Humans are a true tropical animal—an essentially hairless being with sweat glands.
- You are warm-blooded and, through metabolism, are constantly generating heat.
- Your skin is your largest organ, accounting for about 10% of your body's weight; it is the primary organ of thermoregulation.
- You have one of the most sensitive and efficient regulatory mechanisms on the planet for surviving and thriving in the heat; it is designed to keep your brain at a relatively constant temperature.
- You sweat, and the evaporation of water from your skin cools the blood in the skin and, thus, the systemic circulation. Fur-covered mammals and birds pant, which evaporates water out of the airways, thus cooling their blood in the pulmonary circulation.
- You do not survive because of physical prowess but by your mental prowess.
- You have only rudimentary defensive mechanisms to protect you in the cold (e.g. frostbite only numbs us; it does not produce a painful warning).

Numbers for drowning, heat deaths, rabies, and tick bites from the Center of Disease Control. Numbers for cold related deaths from the National Weather Service and Public Health.gov. Numbers for deaths due to hornet/wasp/bee stings, bear attacks, and snake bites from the National park Service. Numbers for lightning deaths from the National Weather Service. Numbers on deaths from spider bites are from 2018 from venemousspiders.net.

Because of these characteristics, humans are perfectly suited to life in the tropics where the ability to shed heat is more important than the ability to retain it. However, as populations grew and moved north or south of the tropics, this ability became a hinderance because they often found themselves cooling off faster than they could generate or maintain heat, resulting in hypothermia, risk of frostbite, and impaired mental function. "A cold brain is a dumb brain."

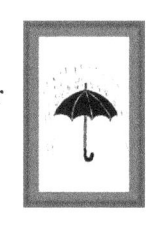

THE HUMAN BRAIN

- In order for your brain to function normally, it needs a constant supply of oxygen and glucose, and a consistent temperature between 97° and 104°F.

- Anatomy and Function: You can think of the brain like an onion with each layer that is added on being a layer of increased function or intelligence.

- The **Brainstem** is at the top of the spinal cord in the center of the brain. It controls the functions that maintain life from second-to-second ("reptilian brain"). Found in this structure are:

  - The respiratory center that controls breathing.
  - The cardiovascular center that controls heart rate and blood pressure.
  - The thermoregulatory center that maintains core temperature.
  - The reticuloactivating center that maintains level of consciousness.

- The **Primitive Brain** or **limbic brain** surrounds the brainstem. It controls the functions that allow you to survive day-to-day and as a species ("primitive brain"):

  - The need to procreate (sex drive).
  - Defensive posturing, primitive aggressive reflexes.

- The **Higher Brain** or **cerebral cortex** is what makes you human. It controls the functions that allow you to survive, strive, and thrive:

  - Gross motor coordination.
  - Fine motor coordination.
  - Reasoning, problem-solving, and judgment.

- When you impair the brain, it loses functions from the most advanced layer, the outermost layer, in. So you lose judgment and problem-solving first and the ability to breathe last.

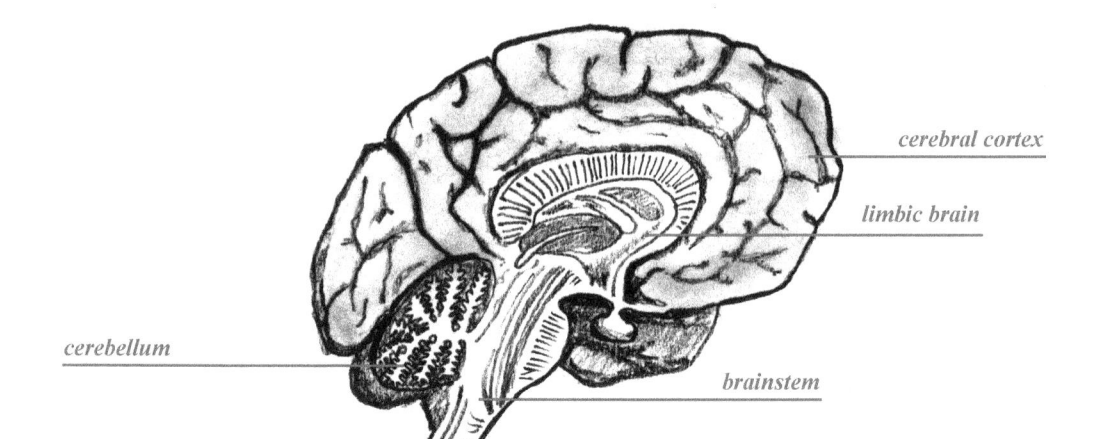

cerebral cortex

limbic brain

cerebellum

brainstem

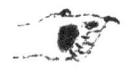

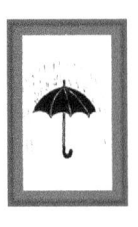

DROWNING

When someone starts to drown they are in a life threat situation, they also present a scene safety problem for rescuers. Someone drowning is in panic mode and can easily overpower and drag down a potential rescuer.

The best plan of action is prevention, make sure the people around you know what behaviors to look for that are typical of someone who is in trouble, and make sure they know what to do if they feel like they themselves are in trouble.

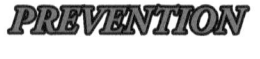 -If you are going to be near water, teach everyone that if they think they are drowning they should flip on their back and float

-Practice this if you have the chance

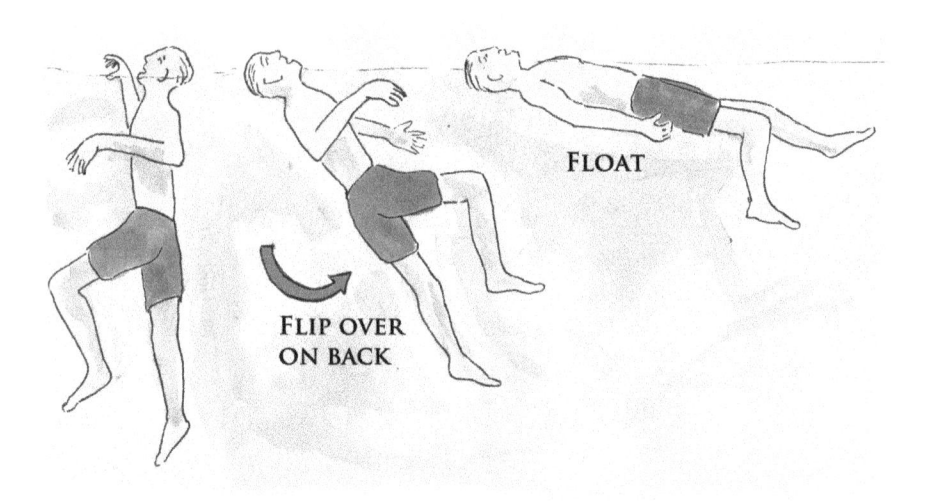

FLOAT

FLIP OVER
ON BACK

What you would see from the shore

The drowning victim will face the shore and reach a hand or hands out of the water

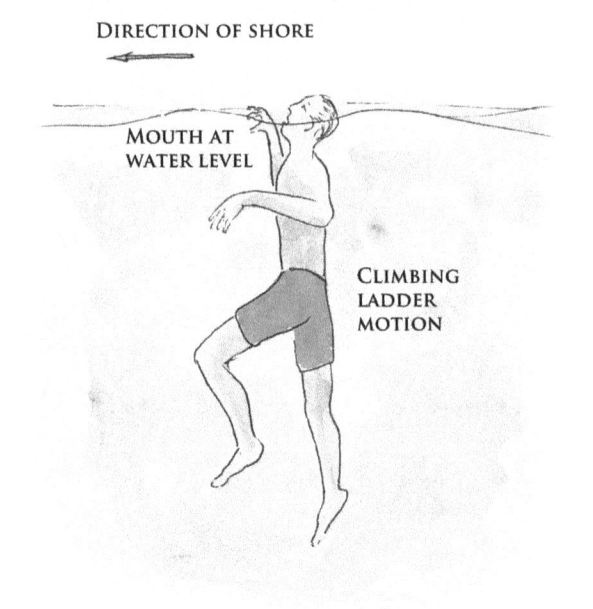

DIRECTION OF SHORE

MOUTH AT
WATER LEVEL

CLIMBING
LADDER
MOTION

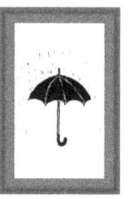

RESCUE PRINCIPLES

Reach, Throw, Row, and Go

Reach: Try and reach the victim with something long and rigid that they can grab

Throw: Try and throw a rope or something that will float to the victim

Row: Try and get to them in a boat
Don't try and get them into the boat, let them hang on

Go: If you cannot Reach, Row, or Throw, you can swim out to help the victim
This is dangerous. A drowning person is panicking and can drag you down too

TREATMENT   *Its the A B Cs....*

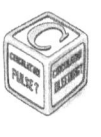

Do they have an **OPEN AIRWAY?** If not, open it.

Are they **BREATHING?**
If not, begin artificial respirations (this can be done while still in the water).
If breaths won't go in, massage throat to relax laryngospasm.
Be prepared for water to come up from the lungs after breaths.

CIRCULATION—do they have a pulse?
If not, begin CPR.
This requires a firm surface.
Expect the patient to vomit during CPR—don't let them aspirate vomitus.

CERVICAL SPINE (inspect, protect if significant MOI
is suspected).

HISTORY (ask bystanders, if available).
How long was the person in the water?
What is the water temperature?
Is the water contaminated? Take a sample.

Is there **RELATED TRAUMA** (e.g., neck injury from diving)?

Treat for **HYPOTHERMIA.**

EVACUATE. Transport all drowning victims, even if fully conscious and coherent, to the local
emergency room for further evaluation and monitoring.

COLD AND HEAT

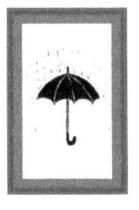

THERMOREGULATION: BALANCING THE TEMPERATURE

HEAT PRODUCTION:

- Basal metabolism is the constant biochemistry that produces heat.
- You burn glucose to produce the heat to drive other chemical reactions.
- Exercise, muscle activity, produces heat.
- Voluntary or involuntary shivering can increase heat production 5x's.

HEAT CONSERVATION:

- Vasoconstriction of the blood vessels in the skin.
- Piloerection—hair standing on end.
- Cessation of sweating.
- Posturing—assuming positions to conserve body heat.

PHYSICS OF HEAT LOSS: (LAWS OF THERMODYNAMICS):

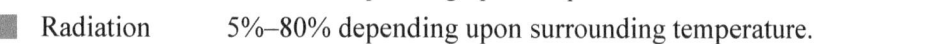

- Conduction   0%–40% depending upon the type of solid material.
- Convection   0%–40% depending upon air penetration.
- Radiation   5%–80% depending upon surrounding temperature.
- Evaporation   0%–90% depending upon vapor pressure & moisture .

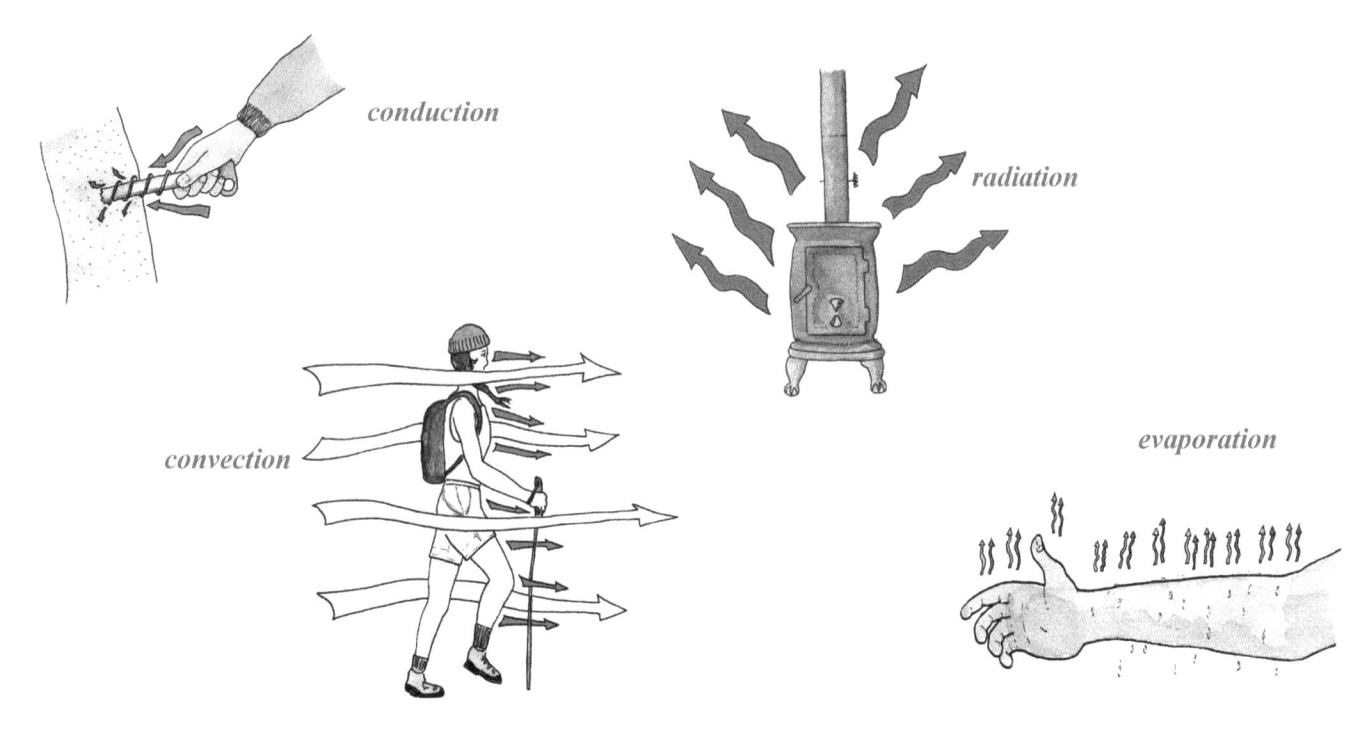

conduction

radiation

convection

evaporation

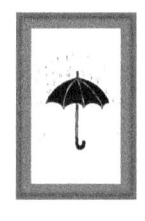

NUTRITION:

Nutritional Requirements: the average person needs about 2500 calories/day.

- Carbohydrate: 4cal/gram 60% (200–400 grams/day = 1200–1600 cal/day).
- Protein: 4cal/gram 30% (30–55 grams/day = 120–220 cal/day).
- Fat: 9cal/gram 10% (20–60 grams/day = 180–540 cal/day).

Number of calories required varies with activity:

- Normal daily activity: 2000–2500 calories/day.
- Winter outdoor sports: 3000–4000 calories/day.
- High altitude activities: 4000–6000 calories/day.

HYDRATION:

Hydration Requirements: the average person needs about two liters of fluid per day.

Normal water losses per day:	Normal Temp	Hot Temp	Heavy Exercise
Skin (moisture loss)	350ml	350ml	350ml
Respiration (breathing)	250ml	350ml	650ml
Sweating	100ml	1400ml	**5000m**
Urination	1400ml	1200ml	500ml
Defecation	100ml	100ml	100ml
TOTALS	2200ml	3400ml	6600ml

Water requirements will vary with activity, sweat output, and altitude.

- Exertional sweat loss is 1–3 liters/hour for up to 4 hours without replacement.
- Altitude has a very low vapor pressure; you will lose about 1cup/hour via respirations.
  (24 cups/24 hrs., 6 quarts or liters/24 hrs., 1½ gallons every 24 hrs.)

You have to be able to make pure potable (drinkable) water.

- If you have to melt snow, you have to know how much fuel to carry.
- Potable water—chemicals, filtering, boiling.

Altitude: we are designed to live between sea level and 8000 feet.

- 8000–14000 feet—the upper limits of sustainable life.
- 14000–18000 feet—high altitude you can visit.
- 18000–28000 feet—very high altitude, constant negative deficit.
- Risk of altitude illness can occur above 5000 feet.
- Risk is increased by rate of ascent. Safe ascent is 1000 feet/day.
- Risk is increased by dehydration, exhaustion, and alcohol consumption.

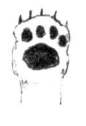

HYPOTHERMIA:

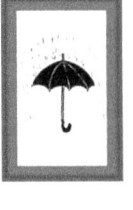

Hypothermia: Is a lowering of the body's core temperature to a level where normal brain & muscle function are impaired. Remember the onion analogy. As the body cools, function is lost from the most advanced layer down.

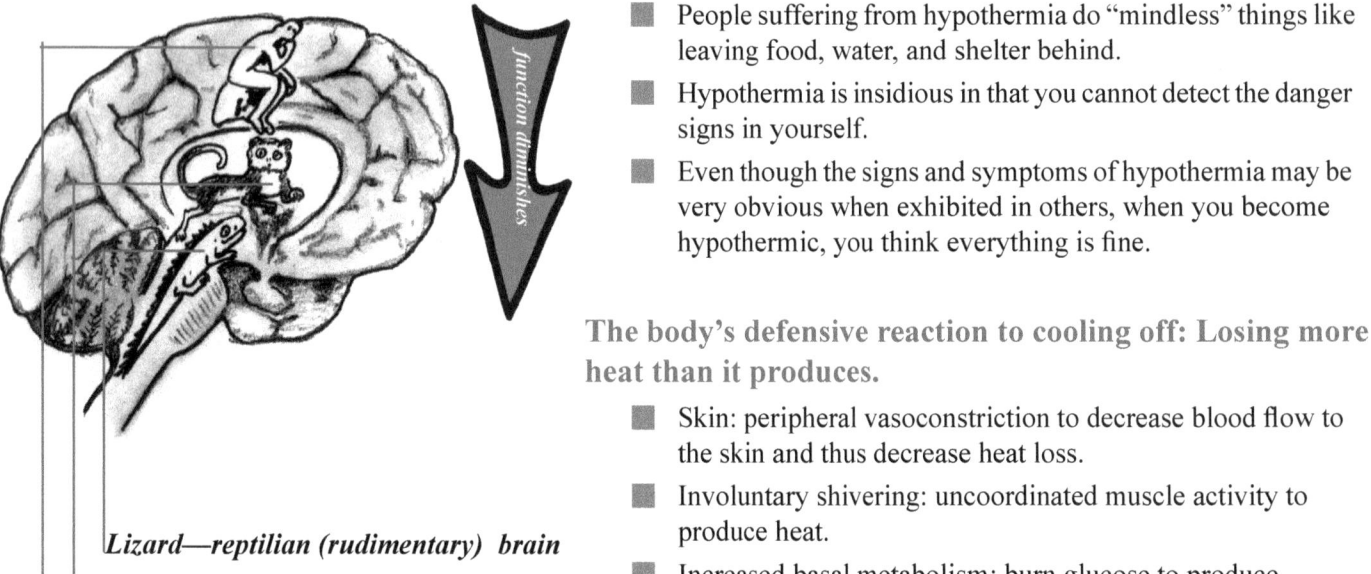

- People suffering from hypothermia do "mindless" things like leaving food, water, and shelter behind.
- Hypothermia is insidious in that you cannot detect the danger signs in yourself.
- Even though the signs and symptoms of hypothermia may be very obvious when exhibited in others, when you become hypothermic, you think everything is fine.

The body's defensive reaction to cooling off: Losing more heat than it produces.

- Skin: peripheral vasoconstriction to decrease blood flow to the skin and thus decrease heat loss.
- Involuntary shivering: uncoordinated muscle activity to produce heat.
- Increased basal metabolism: burn glucose to produce heat—rate may increase 5 fold.
- Behavioral: put on warm clothes, seek out shelter, warmth, protection.

Lizard—reptilian (rudimentary) brain

Lemur—limbic (primitive) brain

Human—cortex (higher) brain

There is no warning of impending doom:

- You do not have a cold center in your brain that warns you that you are becoming hypothermic.
- You get cold, you get dumb, you get lost, you get hurt, you cause problems.

Stages of Hypothermia:

98.6F	Normal
97F	The brain falters, judgment fails, protective & survival instincts decrease. At this point you are in trouble, as you do not take measures to protect yourself. As temperature decreases, mental abilities decrease.
96F	Shivering begins, a constant fine motor tremor. You cannot stop it. It interferes with coordinated muscle activity.
94F	You shiver harder; coordination is failing; you begin tripping and falling.
92F	Shivering is intense; you are unable to walk.
90F	Shivering is convulsive; you assume the fetal position; you are unable to talk.
86F	and below: The "Metabolic Icebox;" you are unconscious, ashen gray; you may appear pulseless and breathless.

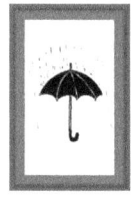

Prevention: **Know your enemy and be prepared for wet, wind, & cold.**

☑ Carry and use rain gear: pants and jacket.

☑ Wear fabrics that stay warm when wet.

☑ Snack often on foods high in quick-burning carbohydrates/glucose.

☑ Stay WELL-HYDRATED.

☑ Carry bivouac gear and know how to use it.

☑ Be attentive to yourself, companions and the environment.

Treatment: **Remove the patient from immediate danger & further exposure.**

☑ Create or seek out shelter.

☑ Get DRY & keep DRY.

☑ Give lots of warm, sweet liquids (JELL-O with <u>sugar</u>) if conscious.

☑ Insulate with hypothermia wrap.

The preferred method for field rewarming of a hypothermic patient involves two principles: Helping the patient to continue to generate body heat and preventing the patient from losing that heat to the environment.

One of the best ways to generate body heat is to feed fuel to the furnace. Foods like powdered JELL-O dissolved in warm water are easy for most patients to take and can provide the needed caloric energy for the patient to start generating more heat.

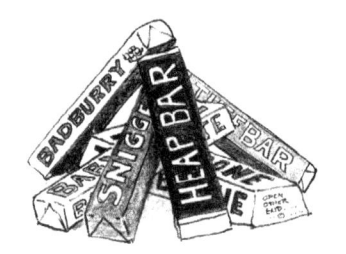

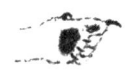

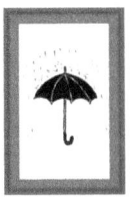

HYPOTHERMIA: THE HYPOWRAP—BUILDING THE HUMAN BURRITO

Once refueling has started, the next step is to stop the patient from losing body heat and create an environment that allows them to store the heat they are producing. The Hypowrap provides an excellent environment for rewarming and protects the patient from the weather.

- Get the patient dry and keep them dry.
- Remove any wet clothing from the patient.
- Reinsulate them with **DRY MATERIAL**—clothing, sleeping bags.
- Place them on an insulating layer such as a dry foam pad.
- Surround the patient with a windproof, waterproof layer—plastic sheeting, tarp.
- Monitor their condition and take appropriate actions as conditions change.

PRINCIPLES OF TREATING HYPOTHERMIA

- Protect from the environment.
- Stop the heat loss.
- Stoke the fire—feed and hydrate.
- Insulate to minimize heat loss.
- If unconscious, do not attempt to feed.
- Make sure everyone in the group is warm and dry.

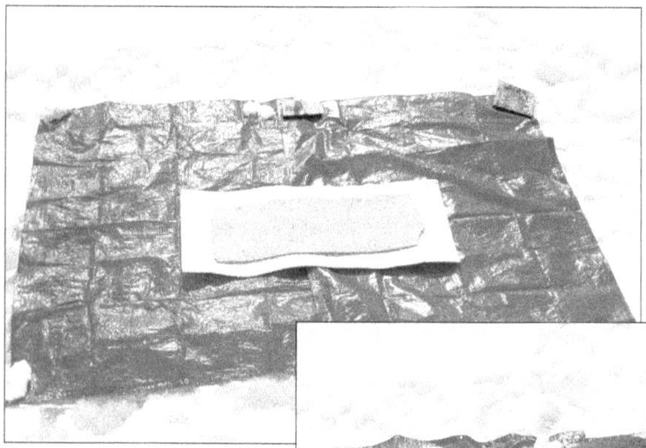

Prepare a base of protective and insulating material. Windproof and waterproof outer layer with insulating layer (ensolite).

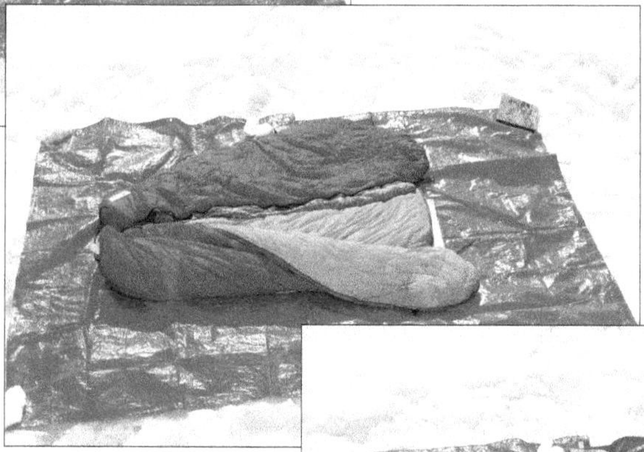

Add lots of dry insulation.

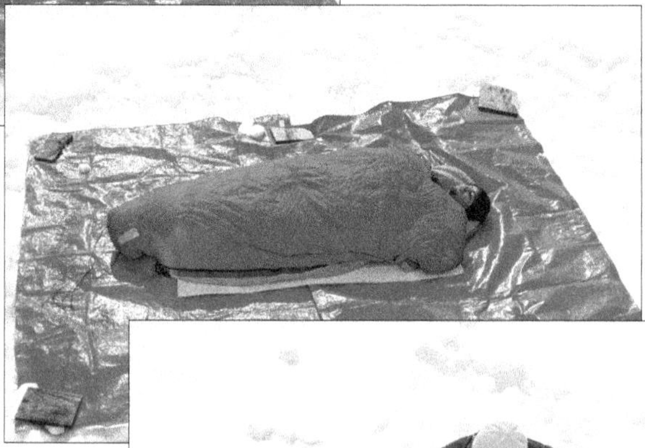

Place patient inside. Double-protect feet and head.

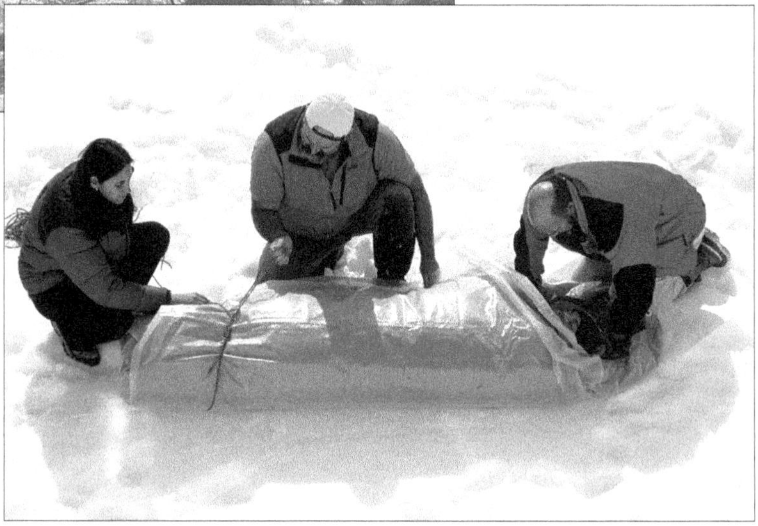

Wrap securely and monitor condition.

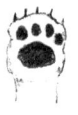

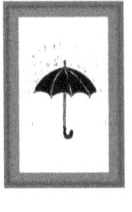

FROSTBITE:

Frostbite: Is a localized cooling and/or freezing of tissue caused by the shunting of blood away from cold areas of the body.

Superficial: description and treatment:

- 1st degree: "frostnip"—numb, soft, cold, pallor.
- 2nd degree: numb, soft, cold, pallor, pain on thawing, and formation of clear fluid-filled or blood-filled bleb.
- Field rewarm using skin-to-skin contact.
- Never massage, rub with snow, or use an external heat source.
- If a bleb forms, protect the area and evacuate the patient.
- Beware of refreezing which can happen quickly and will cause much greater tissue damage.

Deep: description and treatment:

- 3rd degree: numb, cold, white, and rock hard; massive blebs form when thawed; extreme pain during thawing.
- Protect the area and evacuate the patient.
- DO NOT field rewarm (once thawed the area is useless and excruciatingly painful).

1st degree

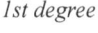

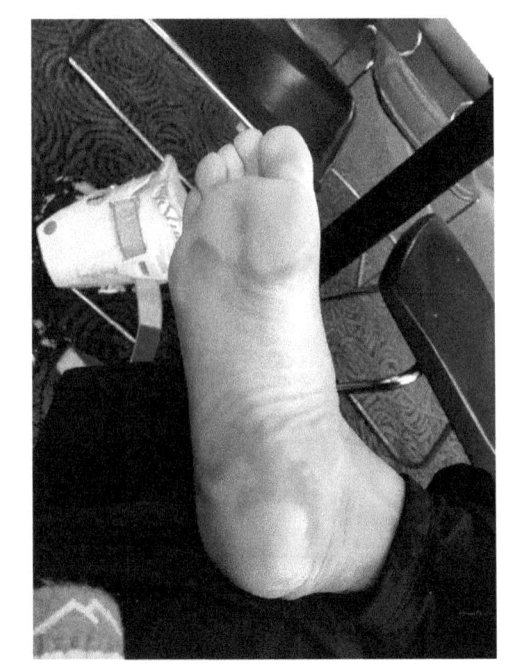

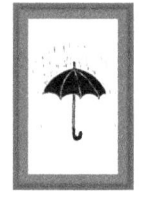

Prevention: Keep the whole body warm.

- ☑ If your feet are cold, put on a hat.

- ☑ Eat & drink to maintain a constant energy/heat production—maintain blood sugar.

- ☑ STAY DRY! CARRY AND USE RAIN GEAR—TOPS & BOTTOMS.

- ☑ Pack extra socks, hats, mittens, or any clothing that is likely to get wet.

- ☑ Wear wool or pile. (Cotton is warm only as long as it is dry.)

- ☑ Do not drink alcohol or use tobacco.

- ☑ Avoid tight clothing, boots, crampons.

- ☑ Keep an eye on each other.

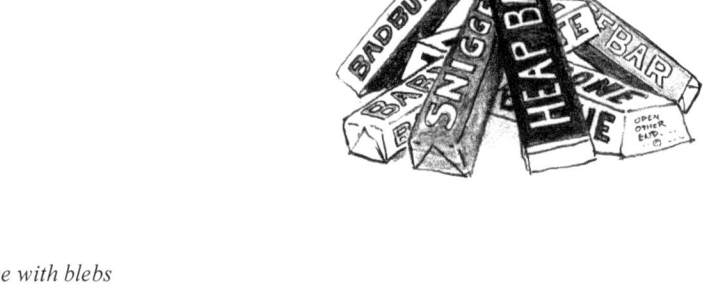

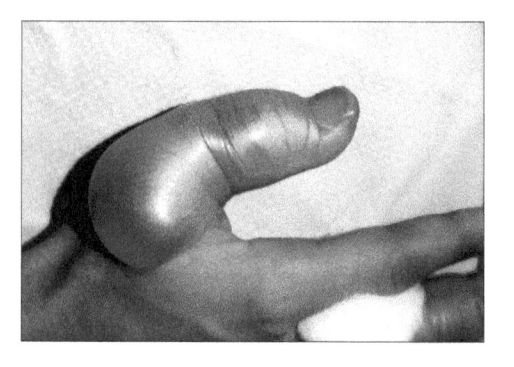

2nd degree with blebs

3rd degree

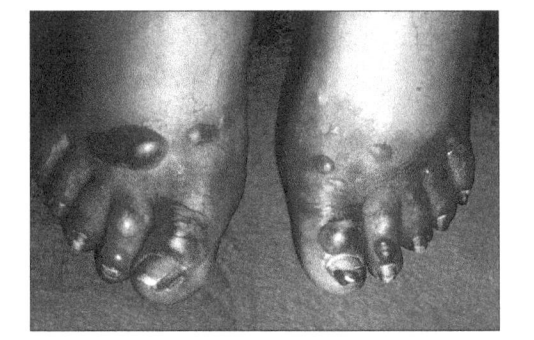

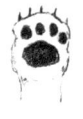

HEAT INJURIES:

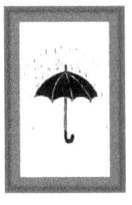

Heat Exhaustion:

- Not a life-threatening emergency. Heat-exhausted patients often recover without care.
- Usually occurs in people who are not acclimatized to heat.
- Cause: A combination of salt and water loss secondary to sweating = dehydration.
- May be associated with heat cramps.
- Heat exhaustion can progress to heat stroke.

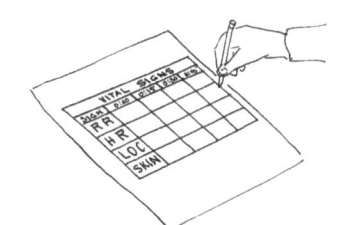

Signs & Symptoms: Typically complain of mild headache, dizziness, and nausea.
- Skin: pale, cool, clammy.
- LOC: may be normal or slightly anxious.
- Pulse: slightly increased, but BP is normal.
- Resp.:   may be normal or slightly increased with normal effort.

Treatment:
- Rest in a cool place in the shade.
- Replace lost fluid & salt—1 teaspoon salt + 8 teaspoons of sugar in 1 liter/quart of water. This is an oral rehydration solution (ORS). ORS can also be used to replace fluids lost from diarrhea, vomiting, fever (sweating), or burns. Other ORS are:
  - Commercial: Gatorade
  - Fruits: oranges, melons, lemons, and limes, either eaten or juiced

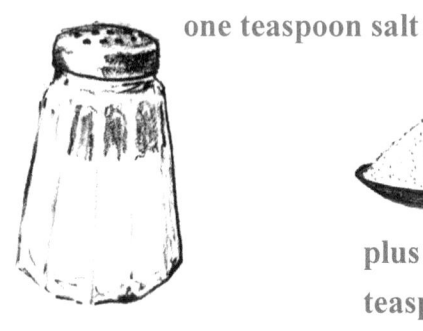

one teaspoon salt

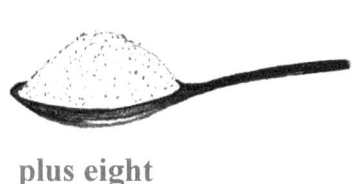

**plus eight
teaspoons sugar**

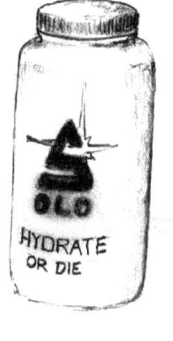

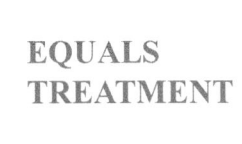

**plus one
liter water**

**EQUALS
TREATMENT**

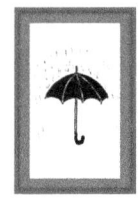

Heat Stroke:

A true LIFE-THREATENING EMERGENCY! The patient will die without immediate care!

Two Causes:
- One: The person has become dehydrated by sweating out fluid faster than they replace it. As their sweating mechanism fails, their body temperature goes up rapidly.
- Two: With a hot day and high humidity, the sweat cannot evaporate off their skin fast enough to cool them. (Exertional heatstroke).

Signs & Symptoms:
- Skin: RED, HOT, DRY (50%); OTHER 50% ARE WET.
- Temp.: 105^0F +, maximum survivable core temperature is 107^0F.
- LOC: Disoriented, confused, combative, hallucinating, eventually coma & death.
- Pulse: Rapid and full; BP may be elevated.
- Resp.:   Full and deep.

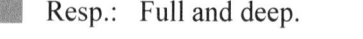

Treatment: This is one of the few conditions where immediate treatment is essential.
- REMOVE FROM HEAT & SUN.
- COOL IMMEDIATELY by soaking with water & fanning to accelerate evaporation.
- Hydrate if possible.
- Vigorously massage limbs.
- Beware of shivering—shivering produces heat.
- Transport immediately to the hospital.

Prevention: Stay out of the hot noonday sun.
- Hydrate or die.
- Stay hydrated & eat salty foods.
- Keep your head covered; wear cotton that will hold moisture which cools the skin.
- Beware of warning signs: feel hot, feel dry, can't pee.

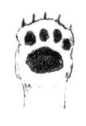

NORTH AMERICAN BITES AND STINGS

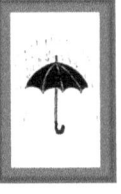

Center for Disease Control Vector-borne Disease Statistics – 2017

TICKBORNE DISEASE CASES PER YEAR – 2017:

Lyme Disease	42,713
Anaplasmosis	7,718
Spotted Fever	6,248
Babesiosis	2,318
Tularemia	239
Powassan	33

MOSQUITO-BORNE DISEASE CASES PER YEAR – 2017

West Nile Virus	2,097
Malaria	2,056 (contracted outside of the US)
Dengue	437 (contracted outside of the US)
Chikungunya	156

Other Environmental Risk Statistics Deaths per year:

Drowning	3,500
Lightning	48 (only 1 out of 7 struck by lightning die)
Hymenoptera	53 (anaphylaxis)
Avalanche	28 (11 in 2017)
Dog Bite	21 (trauma)
Spider Bite	6
Snake Bite	5.2 (7000-8000 people are bitten by snakes each year but only just over 5 bites are fatal

SNAKES

- The primary reason people are bitten by snakes is that they pick them up.
- Bites usually occur on the hand.

Treatment of snake bites:

INSECTS

DO'S ☑ DO CALL 911, seek immediate help

☑ DO KEEP THEM CALM, lay them down and keep them comfortable

☑ DO TRY TO ID THE SNAKE, but do not get bit, one patient is enough

☑ DO REMOVE ANY CONSTRICTING CLOTHING OR JEWELERY, the bite sitand the extremity will swell

☑ DO PLACE THE BITE SITE BELOW THE LEVEL OF THE HEART

☑ DO CONSIDER A PRESSURE IMMOBILIZATION WRAP, but not with a rattlesnake bites (pit vipers – Viperi

☑ DO MONITOR YOUR PATIENT AND MONITOR FOR ANAPHYLAXIS

PRINCIPLES:

Dog Bite or any mammal bite is it: Wound Cleaning →Tetanus Status→Risk of Rabies

Any concern regarding possibility of rabies = vaccination!

Consider this; 4.5 million people are bitten by domestic dogs each year in the U.S., 800,000 of those bite victims require medical treatment.

- Do not pet or put your face near strange dogs.

- Hymenoptera: Bees, Hornets, Wasps, Fire Ants

Signs and Symptoms:
- Pain, local swelling, redness, and itching are common.

Treatment:
- Remove stinger/poison sack by scraping; do not use tweezers.
- Assess and Monitor for anaphylaxis.
- Use topical "bite and sting" stick for comfort.
- Give an oral antihistamine to prevent an allergic reaction: Benadryl (diphenhydramine) 25mg, 2 every 4 hours x 24 hours.

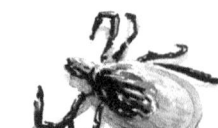

Ticks:

They are tiny septic tanks and carry several infectious diseases.
- Can spread Lyme Disease (the most common, but ticks can carry eight other diseases).
- Small to tiny with large abdomens and short legs.
- Color ranges from tan to brown, almost black.
- They attach to the host, bury their head in the skin, and take a blood meal for a day or more.
- Disease is spread by their saliva, an anticoagulant.

Treatment:
- Remove by pulling off (grasp as close to skin as possible); clean area well.

Mosquitoes and other blood-sucking insects:

- Can be vectors for infectious diseases: Malaria, Equine Enchephalitis, Nile Virus, etc.
- Avoid being bitten by using insect repellents, protective clothing, and sleeping under mosquito netting.

Prevention of tickborne and mosquito-borne diseases:

- Use insect repellents or insecticides.
- The insecticide Permethrin is very effective. It kills the ticks. But it does not adhere well to the skin, so it should be applied to clothing.
- If spraying permethrin onto pants, remember to turn them inside out and spray the inside as well.
  Permethrin can also be used on tents and mosquito netting.

- The insect repellant DEET can be applied directly to the skin. It is a "repellent" and helps to keep the bugs away, but it does not kill them.
- Use DEET with caution on children; it should be less than 30% concentration.

- Wear protective clothing which includes shoes and socks with the long pants tucked into the socks.
  A long sleeve shirt would also be appropriate.

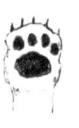

LIGHTNING

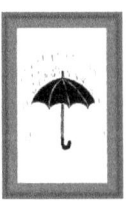

Laws of Nature:

- Lightning can and will do anything. It is unpredictable and uncontrollable.
- Lightning is most likely to strike the highest object around and follow the path of least resistance.

Rules to Live by:

- Thunderstorms are most dangerous as they approach, especially when within 1 mile.
- Don't be the highest object around to avoid a DIRECT STRIKE.
- Stay away from the highest objects to avoid SPLASH or STEP VOLTAGE.
- If on or near water, get off and away from the shoreline.
- Don't sit under overhangs or get into shallow caves.
- Lightning flows like water, so stay out of gullies and washes.
- Calculating Lightning's Distance—Light 286,000 miles/second vs. Sound 700 mph. Count the delay between flash and rumble: 5 seconds = 1 mile.
- Thunderstorms travel at approximately 20-25 mph, e.g. a storm approaching from 3 miles away (15 sec) will be in striking range in 6 minutes.

Places to Avoid or Get off:

- Mountain summits.
- Ridges and cliff tops.
- Overhangs and shallow caves.
- Ditches, gullies, streams.
- Tall trees, poles, large boulders, high objects.
- Open areas, fields, meadows, any place in which you are the highest object.

What to Do If Caught Out:

- ☑ Get off the summit and below tree line if possible.
- ☑ Once below treeline, seek out a low spot among small trees.
- ☑ Stay away from tall trees, cliff faces, and streams.
- ☑ Sit on your pack, pad, or other insulator with your knees flexed, and hug your knees.
- ☑ Keep your feet together to minimize the ground effect of a near-by strike.

Injuries: May Include:

- Respiratory arrest that can progress to cardiac arrest.
- Burns.
- Soft Tissue Injuries.
- Musculoskeletal injuries.

Treatment:

- ☑ Maintain ABCs; closely monitor for respiratory arrest.
- ☑ Do a complete physical exam.
- ☑ Treat all injuries.
- ☑ If conscious, force fluids to help prevent late complications.
- ☑ Evacuate.

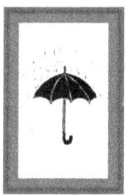

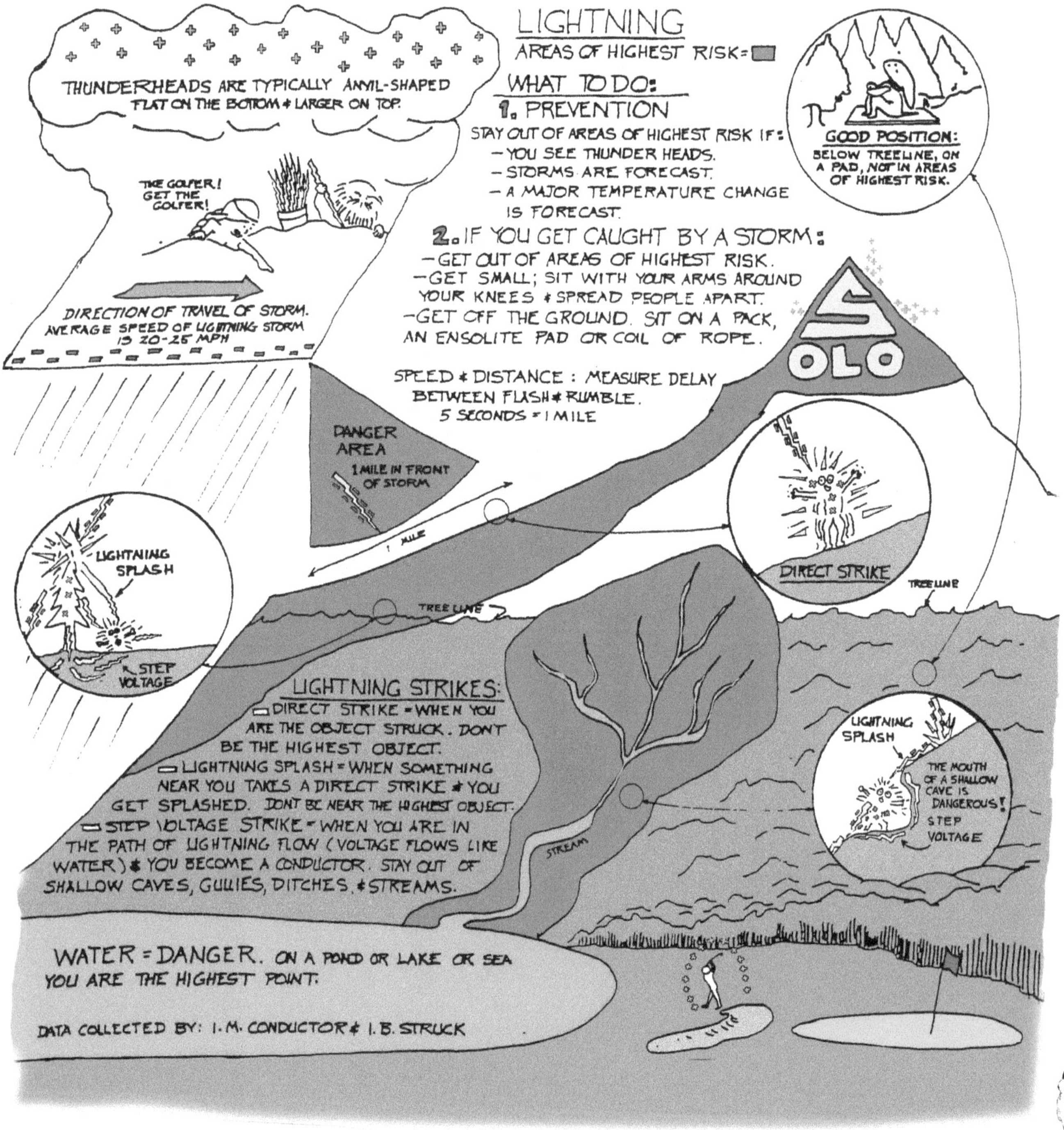

LIGHTNING

AREAS OF HIGHEST RISK = ▨

THUNDERHEADS ARE TYPICALLY ANVIL-SHAPED FLAT ON THE BOTTOM & LARGER ON TOP.

THE GOLFER! GET THE GOLFER!

DIRECTION OF TRAVEL OF STORM. AVERAGE SPEED OF LIGHTNING STORM IS 20-25 MPH

WHAT TO DO:

1. PREVENTION

STAY OUT OF AREAS OF HIGHEST RISK IF:
- YOU SEE THUNDER HEADS.
- STORMS ARE FORECAST.
- A MAJOR TEMPERATURE CHANGE IS FORECAST.

2. IF YOU GET CAUGHT BY A STORM:
- GET OUT OF AREAS OF HIGHEST RISK.
- GET SMALL; SIT WITH YOUR ARMS AROUND YOUR KNEES & SPREAD PEOPLE APART.
- GET OFF THE GROUND. SIT ON A PACK, AN ENSOLITE PAD OR COIL OF ROPE.

SPEED & DISTANCE : MEASURE DELAY BETWEEN FLASH & RUMBLE. 5 SECONDS = 1 MILE

GOOD POSITION: BELOW TREELINE, ON A PAD, NOT IN AREAS OF HIGHEST RISK.

S OLO

DANGER AREA
1 MILE IN FRONT OF STORM

1 MILE

LIGHTNING SPLASH

STEP VOLTAGE

TREE LINE

DIRECT STRIKE

TREE LINE

LIGHTNING SPLASH

THE MOUTH OF A SHALLOW CAVE IS DANGEROUS! STEP VOLTAGE

STREAM

LIGHTNING STRIKES:
☐ DIRECT STRIKE = WHEN YOU ARE THE OBJECT STRUCK. DON'T BE THE HIGHEST OBJECT.
☐ LIGHTNING SPLASH = WHEN SOMETHING NEAR YOU TAKES A DIRECT STRIKE & YOU GET SPLASHED. DON'T BE NEAR THE HIGHEST OBJECT.
☐ STEP VOLTAGE STRIKE = WHEN YOU ARE IN THE PATH OF LIGHTNING FLOW (VOLTAGE FLOWS LIKE WATER) & YOU BECOME A CONDUCTOR. STAY OUT OF SHALLOW CAVES, GULLIES, DITCHES, & STREAMS.

WATER = DANGER. ON A POND OR LAKE OR SEA YOU ARE THE HIGHEST POINT.

DATA COLLECTED BY: I. M. CONDUCTOR & I. B. STRUCK

THE BACKCOUNTRY ESSENTIALS:

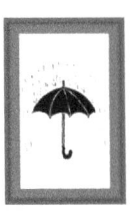

ATTITUDE: THINK POSITIVELY.

- Positive attitude: belief that you can always make things better.
- Will to survive.

FOOD: GET FUEL TO BURN.

- High carbohydrate foods that require no preparation & provide quick energy.
- High carbohydrate foods that can be made into a warm drink (Jello).

WATER: QUENCH YOUR THIRST.

- Minimum of 2 liters per day if not active (up to 1-3 liters/hour if active).
- The ability to disinfect water (chemicals, filtering, boiling).

CLOTHING: STAY WARM & DRY.

- Warm clothing that retains heat even when wet (spare socks & hat).
- Waterproof rain gear, both tops and bottoms (large garbage or leaf bags).

SHELTER: GET DRY & STAY DRY.

- Ability to improvise shelter (10' x 10' plastic sheet, p-cord, space blanket).
- Comfort & light (plumber's candles).

FIRE: GET WARM.

- Ability to build a fire (waterproof matches, tinder, candles).
- Ability to make kindling (pocket knife).
- Ability to warm water (tin cup).

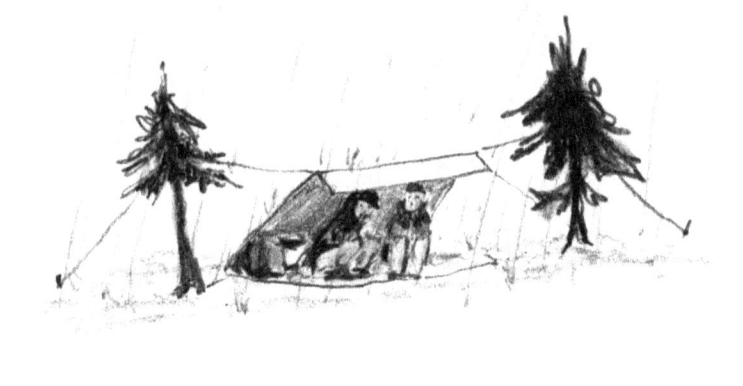

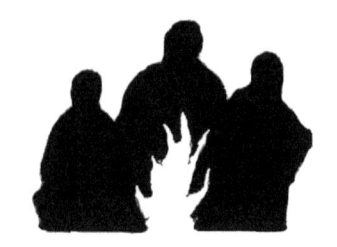

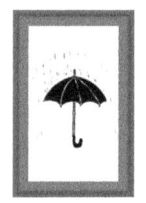

NAVIGATION: KNOW WHERE YOU'RE GOING.

- Map & Compass; know how to use them.
- Ability to find your way at night (route-finding skills and flashlight).

WEATHER: KNOW THE ENVIRONMENT.

- Basic understanding of weather patterns.
- Knowledge of how to react to severe weather, lightning, etc.

SIGNALING: GET HELP.

- Whistle (preferably plastic) and signal mirror (whistle and/or mirror).

EXPERIENCE: PRACTICE SURVIVAL SKILLS BEFORE YOU NEED THEM.

- The most valuable and versatile survival tool is between your ears.

AVOID THE SURVIVAL SITUATION:

☑ Make a plan and work the plan.

☑ Know your limitations and the group's limitations.

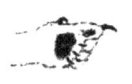

BIVUOAC & SURVIVAL SKILLS:

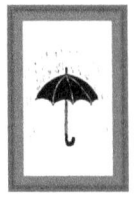

CRISIS INTERVENTION:

☑ Be prepared to bivouac.

☑ Keep everyone warm and dry.

☑ Know how to get help.

☑ Send out two for help.

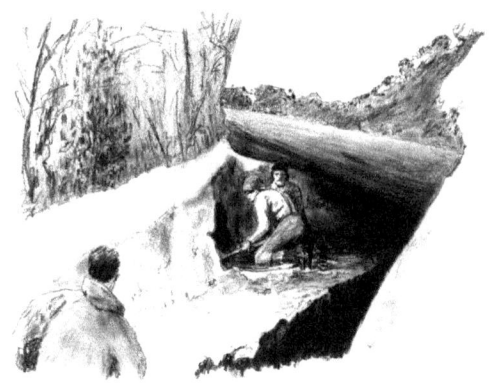

☑ Send out a SOAPnote.
- ■ Send out your group's ability to stay put.
- ■ Send out a map with your exact location marked on it.
- ■ Know how to build a fire and make yourself very big, easy to find (surveyor's tape).

Factors that contribute to a crisis:

☑ Fatigue, taking on too much.

☑ Pushing hard or rushing to get someplace.

☑ Weather.

☑ Equipment failure or, more often, the wrong equipment.

☑ Lack of equipment.

☑ Personality problems.

☑ Poor judgment, making wrong decisions for wrong reasons—ego.

IF YOU WANT TO BE FOUND:

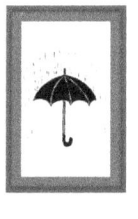

☑ "Hug a tree" - Stay put, don't wander around.

☑ Make yourself big and obvious:
- Build a smoky fire.
- Put out long pieces of brightly colored surveyor's tape.
- Mark the area with broken branches, clothing.

BIVOUAC KIT: THE 16 ESSENTIALS FOR YOUR BACKPACK:

Best option—Carry a "bivy kit" in a stuff sack:
- Spare hat—balaclava; can cover your whole face and neck.
- Spare socks—for feet and can also act as emergency mittens.
- Space blanket or big garbage/leaf bag.
- Metal cup—that you can hold over a candle or fire to melt snow.
- JELL-O—with real sugar.
- Hard candies—with real sugar.
- Plumber's candles—short, thick, and long-burning.
- Waterproof matches—some people like to also carry a lighter.
- Compass.
- Whistle and/or signaling mirror.
- Knife.
- Parachute cord—100".
- Surveyor's tape—bright color.
- Plastic 6 mil or tarp—10' x 10'.
- Paper and pencil.
- Duct tape.

Bivouac Skills: What to do with what you have:

Improvised shelters—bivouacs:
- Severe weather bivouac—"bombproof."
- Lean-to—roomy, but easily blown apart.
- Worst option: Just you, "WHAT IF!" NO FOOD, NO WATER, NO SHELTER?

No snow—debris piles:
- Large overhanging trees.
- Overhangs & caves.

Snow—snow piles = Quinzee:
- Snow trenches.
- Snow caves.
- Large evergreens with branches close to the ground.

— *NOTES* —

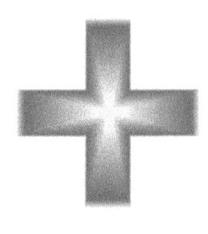

CHAPTER FOUR

SOFT TISSUE INJURIES
&
MEDICAL EMERGENCIES
From Minor Wounds to Critical Care

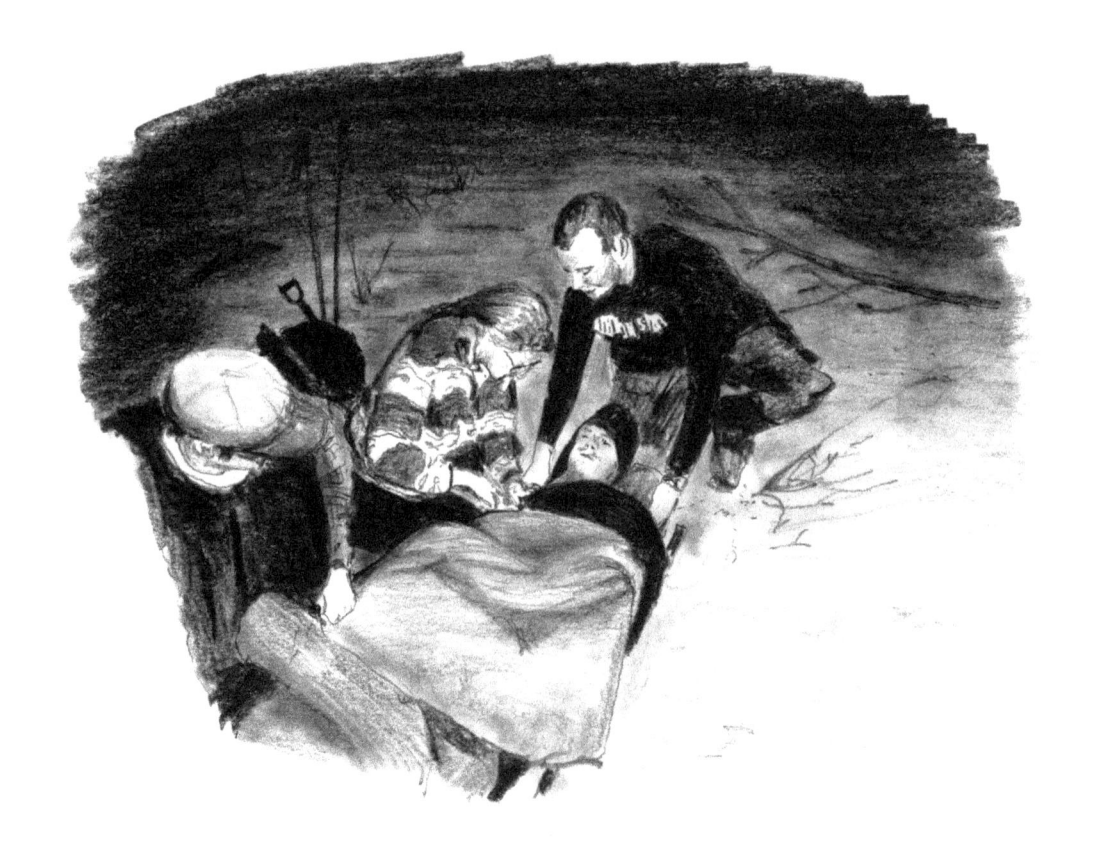

SOFT TISSUE INJURIES:

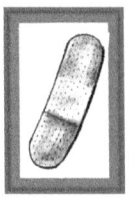

SOFT TISSUES:

- Everything except the bones.
- This section concentrates on insults and injuries to the skin and structures immediately under the skin: fat, muscles, & blood vessels.

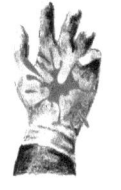

Remember: Total Body Fluid Precautions—BSI

THE PIPES: ARTERIES, VEINS, & CAPILLARIES

They are muscular tubes that expand and contract depending on required blood flow.

- Arteries are the blood vessels leaving the heart.
  - They are under pressure: the systolic blood pressure—100 to 120 mmHg
  - Arteries are deep, protected, lying under the muscles directly on top of the bones.
  - When arteries are cut, they spurt like little oil wells—this is very rare.
- Veins are the blood vessels returning to the heart.
  - They are under very little pressure—10 to 20 mmHg pressure.
  - Veins are superficial and can be seen and felt under the skin.
  - When veins are cut, they drain blood. How much depends on the diameter of the vein.
- Capillaries are the tiny blood vessels that carry oxygen to the cells.
  - They are microscopic.
  - They are the most abundant vessels in the body.
  - One pound of body tissue has 1 mile of capillaries.
  - Capillaries in the skin expand and contract to control blood flow to the skin.
  - When cut, they seep or ooze blood

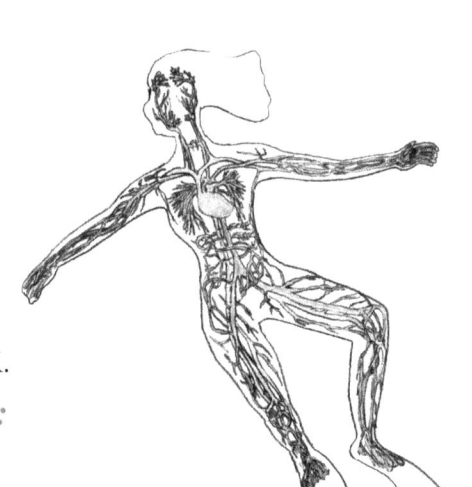

THE LIQUID: BLOOD—"THE RED STUFF"

- Carries oxygen, nutrients, and water to all the cells of the body.
- Carries away carbon dioxide and waste products.
- Carries heat into the extremities.
- Loss of blood causes a potentially life-threatening condition—SHOCK.

PRINCIPLES OF MANAGING SOFT TISSUE INJURIES:

- Control Bleeding
- Clean
- Bandage
- Monitor

TO CONTROL BLEEDING:

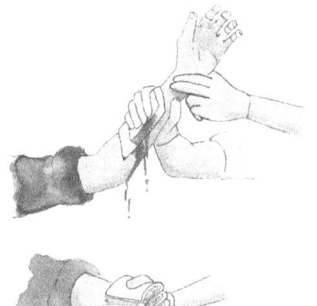
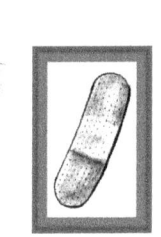

☑ Direct Pressure:
- ▣ Apply pressure directly over the wound and compress to stop the bleeding.
- ▣ Maintain pressure for about 10 minutes.

☑ Pressure Dressing:
- ▣ To maintain constant pressure, place something bulky and absorbent over the wound, an inch or two thick.
- ▣ Wrap the dressing with an elastic bandage for about 10 minutes.
- ▣ Then loosen the dressing to ensure circulation distal to the injury.
- ▣ Once bleeding has been controlled for 20–30 minutes, direct pressure can be stopped so the wound can be inspected and properly cleaned.

WOUND PACKING

- ▣ For a life-threatening bleed where a tourniquet can not be used, pack the wound with bleeding control gauze (hemostatic gauze), plain gauze, or a clean cloth and then apply pressure with both (gloved) hands.
- ▣ Apply steady pressure with both hands directly on top of the bleeding wound. Press down hard on the bleeding would and continue to press down.

BUT WHAT IF...

If unable to control bleeding with direct pressure:
- ▣ Apply tourniquet two to three inches above the injury.

Improvised Tourniquet

1. Wrap a wide band around the extremity, not over clothing, at least 2" to 3" proximal to the bleeding and not over the elbow or knee.

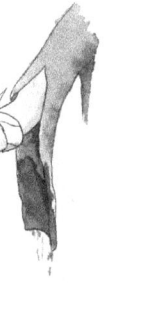

2. Tie a simple knot in the band.

3. Place a 6" stick or bar over the knot and tie a second knot over it to secure it.

4. Using the stick as a "Spanish windlass," twist it to tighten the band.

5. Tighten the windlass until both the bleeding and the distal pulse stop.

6. Secure the free end of the windlass in place with another band or tape.

7. Write a capital "T" and the time of application on the patient's forehead.

8. If possible, cold pack the extremity to increase the duration of survivability, just like an amputation.

9. Evacuate immediately.

Locate the tourniquet above, or proximal, to the injury.

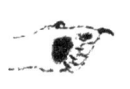

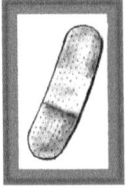

SPECIFIC SOFT TISSUE INJURIES:

Contusions:

- Bruises: mild swelling, discoloration, may be painful.

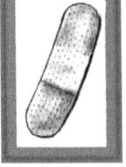

- ☑ Rest, Ice, Compression, and Elevation (RICE) to limit swelling.

- ☑ Protect and watch injury closely in cold weather as it will freeze quicker than usual.

Abrasions:

- Scrapes may be painful, dirty, and can easily become infected.

- ☑ Very little bleeding; while wound is pain-free, scrub thoroughly with soap & water

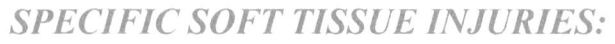

- ☑ Allow to air dry before bandaging.

- ☑ You may apply antibiotic ointment for comfort.

Lacerations/Incisions:

- May bleed profusely or require pressure dressing.

- ☑ Control bleeding and maintain hemostasis for 20–30 minutes.

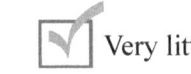

- ☑ Cleanse well with copious irrigation.

- ☑ For large gaping wound—control bleeding, cleanse, approximate edges, don't close tightly.

- 🚫☑ If stitched or butterflied closed, infection is likely. It may have to be re-opened.

Flap Avulsion:

- Three-sided tear, one side still attached.

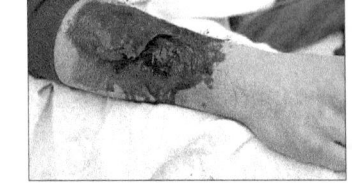

- ☑ Control bleeding; then rinse under flap with water, and bandage it in its anatomical position.

Amputation:

◼ A body part is completely severed.

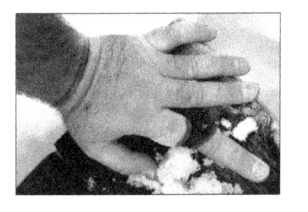 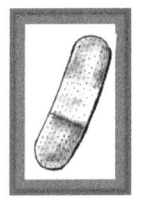

   ✓ Wrap the part in a moist sterile dressing, and seal it in a plastic bag.

   ✓ Immerse the bag in ice water, and evacuate both the patient and the part to the hospital.

Punctures:

◼ Small penetrating wound to the skin.

   ✓ Gently irritate to cause some bleeding to flush out the wound.

   ✓ Monitor for infection; this is the wound most likely to become infected.

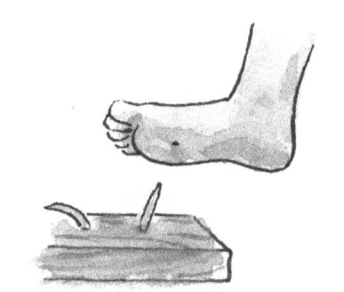

Impaled Objects:

◼ Something stuck in the body that doesn't belong there.

   ✓ Use common sense; if easily removed, remove it.

   ✓ Once removed, use direct pressure to control bleeding..

◼ Impaled object may be removed if:

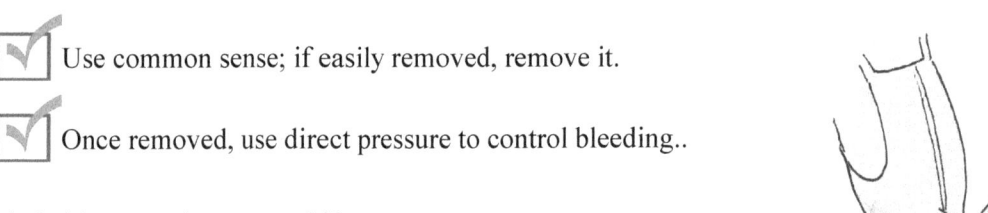

   ✓ It is in an extremity.

   ✓ It is in the cheek of the face (or buttocks).

   ✓ It is metal in a cold environment.

   ✓ It is too large or hard to cut off.

◼ Do not remove impaled objects if: (These objects should be bandaged in plac

   ◼ In the skull or neck.
   ◼ In the chest, possibly into the lungs.
   ◼ In the abdomen, possibly penetrating.

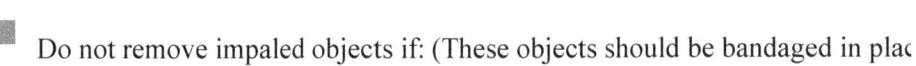

◼ What about fish hooks?

   ✓ Easily removed by pushing away from the barb and backing out.

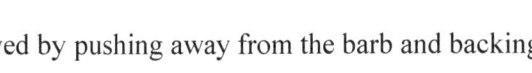 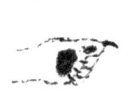

SOFT TISSUE INJURIES:

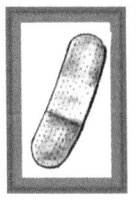

LONG-TERM WOUND CARE—DEFINITIVE CARE IS LONGER THAN 24 HOURS AWAY:

Prevent infection and promote healing by:

■ Properly cleaning the wound—once bleeding has been controlled for 20-30 minutes:

☑ Remove dressings and closely inspect the wound.

☑ Check circulation, sensation, and motion (CSM) distal to the injury.

☑ Debride, remove any foreign material in the wound like sticks, grass, etc.

☑ Clean around the wound with soap & water or with a dilute solution of iodine.

☑ Clean the wound by irrigation with a forceful flow of sterile water or a dilute solution of iodine by using an irrigation syringe or water bottle.

☑ Cover the wound with dry sterile dressings and keep clean & dry.

☑ Bandage the sterile dressings in place.

☑ Change the dressings every 12 hours, and examine the wound for signs of infection.

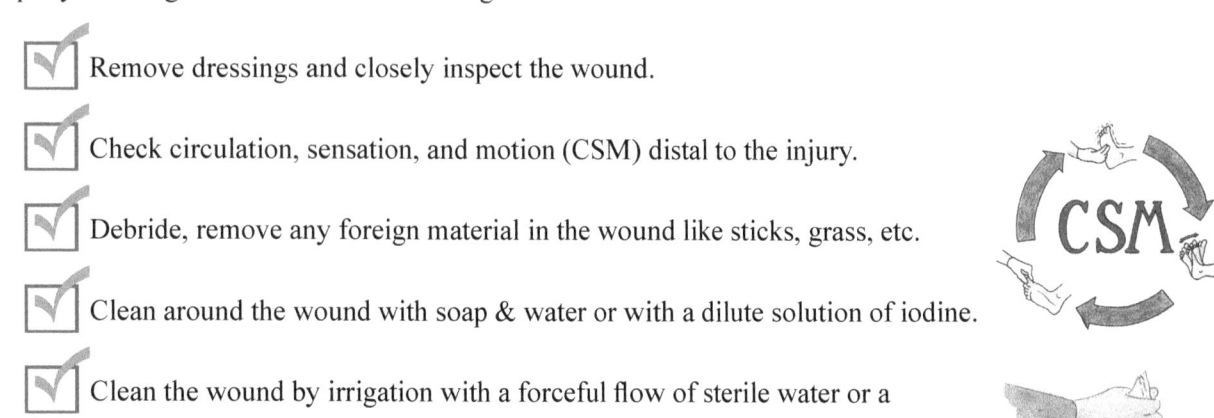

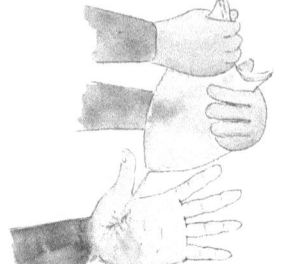

But what if...

■ If the wound is dirty or unable to be kept clean and dry:

☑ Cover the wound with a dressing soaked with a dilute solution of iodine, less than 2% strength.

☑ Change every 6 hours.

■ There is impaired CSM distal to the injury:

☑ Do all of the above.

☑ Then splint.

☑ Then evacuate.

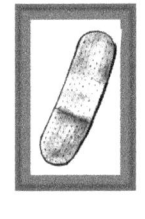

WOUND CARE DO'S AND DON'TS:

DO'S

 Protect from further injury, freezing, and from contamination by proper bandaging.

DON'TS

 Don't tightly close a wound with butterfly bandages or suturing.

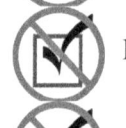 Don't fill the wound with an antibiotic ointment.

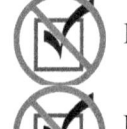 Don't leave a pressure dressing in place for more than 20 minutes.

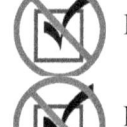 Don't allow the wound to freeze.

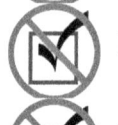 Don't be afraid of causing pain to properly clean a wound.

WHEN SHOULD YOU EVACUATE FOR STITCHES?

- If the cut goes through the skin (causes gaping) and is longer than 1 inch—cosmetic repair.
- If the cut is in the face, hands, or over a joint.
- If there is an injury to a nerve, ligament, or tendon.
- Check for distal CIRCULATION, SENSATION, and MOTION.

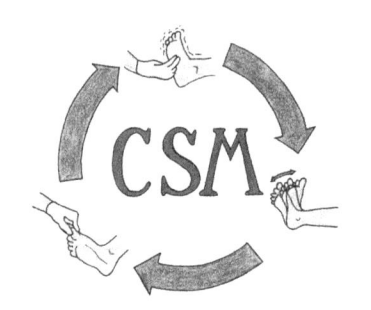

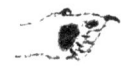

73

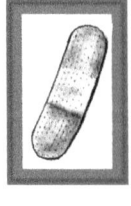

INFECTIONS:

- ▪ Caused by contamination of the wound by bacteria.
- ▪ Bacteria want to be warm, moist, and in the dark.
- ▪ Bacteria double (reproduce) every 30 minutes at 98°F (37°C).
- ▪ Signs and symptoms of an infection are a result of your immune system's response to the invading bacteria.
- ▪ Risk of tetanus; know shot status (good for ten years).

Rapid Reproduction of Bacteria		
No. of Bacteria	*Elapsed Hours*	
1	*0*	*—*
16	*2*	*tens*
256	*4*	*hundreds*
1,024	*5*	*thousands*
131,072	*8.5*	*hundreds of thousands*
1,048,376	*10*	*millions*
1,073,537,024	*15*	*billions*
1,024,000,000,000	*20*	*trillions*
256,000,000,000,000	*24*	*256 trillion hungry little mouths to feed*

Signs of infection:

Early: localized to the skin and wound area:
- ▪ Red (rubor)—due to dilated capillary beds, increased blood flow to the area.
- ▪ Warm (calor)—due to the increased blood flow.
- ▪ Swollen (tumor)—due to the increased blood flow.
- ▪ Tender (dolor)—due to swelling.

Late—severe potentially life-threatening:
- ▪ Pus formation—collection of white blood cells, may be draining from the wound.
- ▪ Streaking up the extremity—due to infection traveling up lymphatics.
- ▪ Swollen and tender lymph nodes—the infection has reached the lymph nodes.
- ▪ Fever and Chills—a sign that the infection is spreading systemically, septic shock.

Treatment of skin infections:

☑ Apply moist heat packs; if possible, soak in hot water with salt.

☑ If the wound is closed but swollen, gently open so it can drain.

☑ Evacuate as soon as possible if red streaks and/or fever develop.

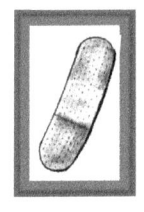

BURNS

THERMAL BURNS

Treatment: get the heat out:

☑ Remove clothing over and around the burn site.

☑ Cool with cold water for at least 15 minutes.

Superficial: First & Second Degree Burns:

■ Appearance: area of the burn will turn red and may form blisters, but the patient has full sensation.

☑ Cold soak the burn with water for 15 minutes.

☑ Protect with a moist sterile dressing.

☑ Evacuate if the burn area is more than the size of their palm.

☑ If the burn area is large and painful, cover with moist dressings for comfort during evacuation.

Deep: Third Degree

■ Appearance: area of the burn may be red, white, charred, blistered, but there is no sensation; the burn is deep enough to destroy the sensory nerves.

☑ All deep burns must be evacuated.

☑ Cold soak the burn with water for 15 minutes.

☑ Cover with a moist dressing and waterproof bandage to prevent evaporation.

☑ Hydrate—force fluids as burns can cause severe dehydration.

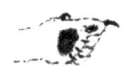

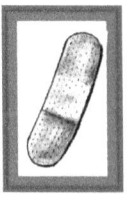

BLISTERS:

- Caused by friction against the skin forcing the layers of the skin apart.
- Common causes are a loose boot or shoe rubbing against the heel, or a shovel handle or oar-loom rubbing against the palms of the hands.
- The body reacts to the abuse by secreting water into the area of trauma.
- Blisters start out as a "hot spot" that, if left unattended to, will grow into a water-filled blister or bleb.

Treatment:

- React to the pain or "hot spot."

  - ☑ If on the foot, remove the sock and boot and apply athletic tape over the hot spot.

  - ☑ Then redress the foot paying attention to how the sock and boot fit.

- If a fluid-filled blister has formed, properly treat and protect the blister.

  - ☑ Clean the area around the blister.

  - ☑ Drain the blister by making small holes around the base with a sterile needle, and gently compress the blister to force out the fluid.

  - ☑ Surround the blister with padding, moleskin, molefoam, Spenco Second Skin, etc.

  - ☑ Fill the well created by the blister dressing with an antibiotic ointment to protect the fragile skin and minimize friction.

  - ☑ Cover the blister area and padding with tape.

  - ☑ If on the foot, redress the foot.

  - ☑ Clean daily and monitor for signs of infection.

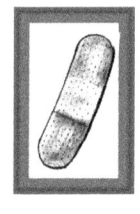

PREVENTION:

- Sock combination—thin on skin, thick over
- Properly fit boots—break them in
- React early to pain or hot spots
- Keep feet dry—wet feet blister easily and quickly

*hot
spot*

blister

*clean, puncture
and deflate*

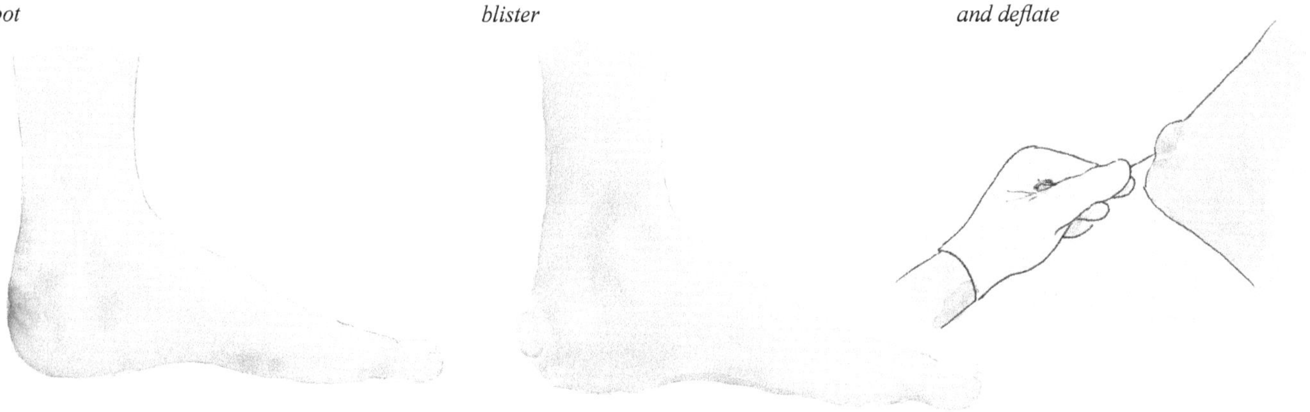

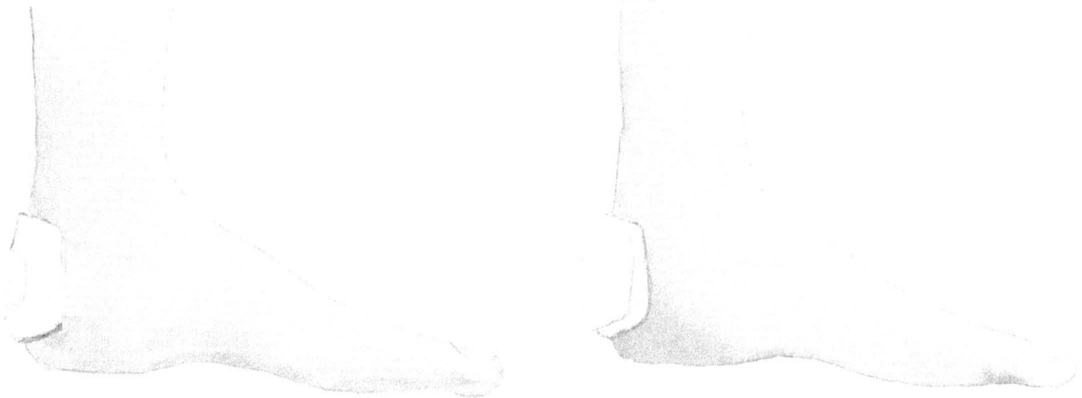

*protect with donut
padding;fill donut
hole with antibiotic
ointment*

*protect and
cover*

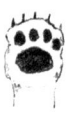

SOFT TISSUE INJURIES:

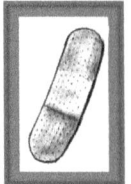

BANDAGING SKILLS:

Dressing: Sterile material put directly onto a wound site.

■ Sterile gauze pads: 2" x 2" or 4" x 4" trauma dressings.

Bandage: Piece of material that holds the dressings in place.

■ Cravat: A large triangular piece of material that is used in very clever ways to hold dressings.

■ ACE bandage: Elastic material 2" to 6" wide that can be used to hold dressings and also to apply compression.

■ Roller gauze/ Kling: Soft, fluffy material in a roll, 1" to 6" wide that can be wrapped to hold a dressing in place.

Specific Bandages:

■ **Scalp bandage**: To hold a dressing on the scalp.

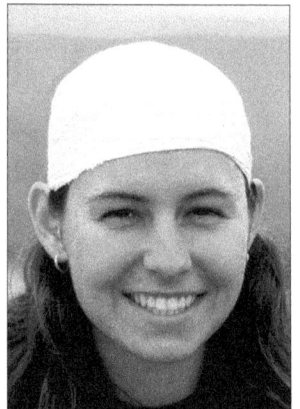

■ **Temporal/Jaw**: To hold a dressing on the side of the head, or to support the jaw.

■ **Shoulder**: To hold a dressing on the shoulder or upper arm and maintain range of motion.

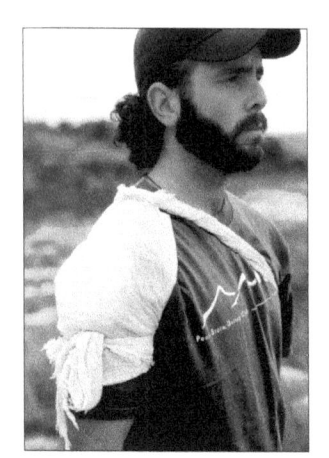

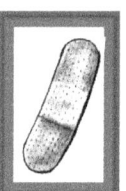

Arm sling & swathe: To support the shoulder, upper arm, elbow, forearm, or wrist.

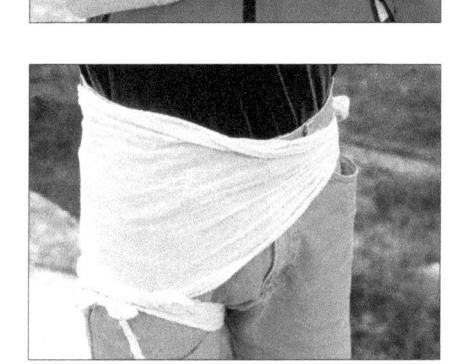

Hip: To hold a dressing on the hip or buttocks and maintain full range of motion of the hip.

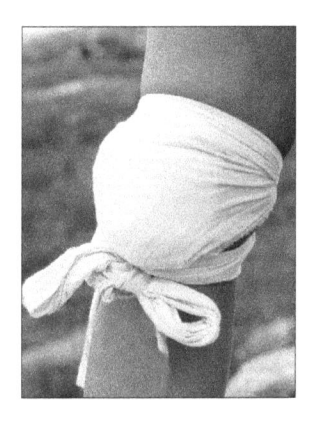

Knee: To hold a dressing on the knee and maintain full range of motion.

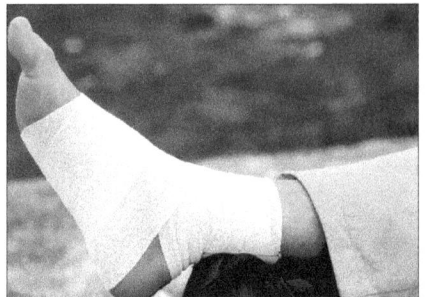

Sprained ankle: RICE
(If needed, use the ankle bandage shown in the Musculoskeletal chapter.)

MEDICAL EMERGENCIES & CRITICAL CARE:

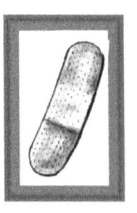

These are rare but potentially life-threatening problems you need to be able to recognize and manage. A good history will usually make the diagnosis.

CHANGE IN LEVEL OF CONSCIOUSNESS:

Level of Consciousness (LOC) is maintained by the brain, so any change indicates a brain problem. Signs and Symptoms:

- ☑ Change in personality.

- ☑ Deteriorating LOC, **A > V > P > U > Death**

- ☑ Seizure activity.

Causes: Your brain needs four things to survive and thrive; causes of change in LOC:

- ☑ Oxygen (hypoxia).

- ☑ Carbohydrates (glucose, hypo/hyperglycemia).

- ☑ Proper temperature, 98.6⁰F/37⁰C (hypo/hyperthermia

- ☑ Proper pressure = intracranial pressure (ICP).

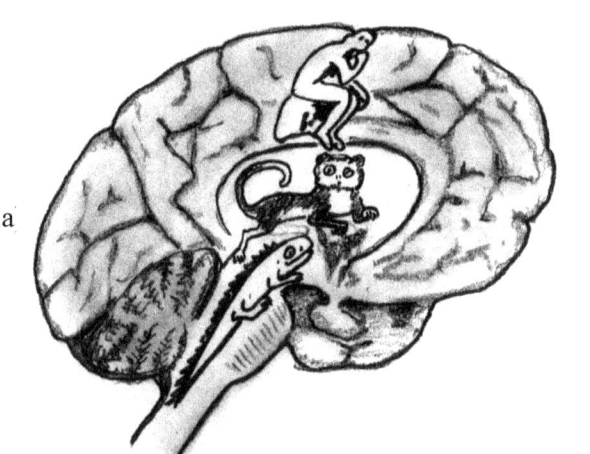

Principles of Management

- ☑ Maintain and monitor the airway & breathing.

- ☑ Place in the Recovery Position to protect the airway.

- ☑ If respiratory rate less than 10 or greater than 30, assist breathing—1 breath every 5 seconds.

- ☑ Recognize the problem early and evacuate early as these problems tend to steadily deteriorate.

- ☑ If suspicious of a diabetic emergency, give them sugar.

- ☑ Get help; this patient needs to be evacuated ASAP.

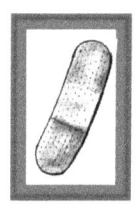

SHORTNESS OF BREATH (SOB)—AIRWAY, BREATHING:

- The brain perceives that it is not getting enough oxygen so it causes a sensation of SOB.
- So, either there is not enough oxygen getting into the blood, or there is not enough oxygenated blood getting to the brain.

Signs and Symptoms:

- Complaining of shortness of breath.
- Rapid shallow or deep breathing.
- Skin color pale to cyanotic (blue) as hypoxia increases.
- May be wheezing.

Causes:

- Lungs: asthma (wheezing).
- Lungs: pneumothorax (no breath sounds on one side)
- Lungs: pulmonary edema, pneumonia (crackles).
- Lungs: pulmonary emboli (dyspnea).
- Heart: MI, angina (chest pain).
- Anaphylaxis, anxiety, altitude.

Principles of Management:

☑ **Look:** is your patient struggling to breathe—mouth open, obvious effort. Are they cyanotic; do they have hives?

☑ **Listen** to the breath sounds: is there wheezing, gurgling, or no breath sounds on one side?
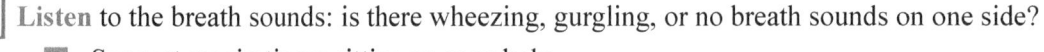
- Support respirations; sitting up may help.
- Assist breathe for them if they cannot move enough air on their own.
- If asthmatic, may use **<u>THEIR</u>** rescue inhaler: Albuterol Metered Dose Inhaler (MDI), 2 puffs every 10 minutes until breathing improves (up to 4 times), then 2 puffs every 4 hours.

☑ If yes to these symptoms, get help—this patient needs to be evacuated **ASAP**.

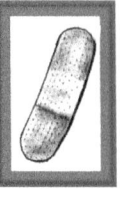

ASTHMA

Allergens in the airway cause swelling, bronchospasm, and increased mucous production in the bronchioles. This causes the bronchioles to narrow resulting in wheezing, air trapping, and shortness of breath.

Signs and Symptoms:

- Shortness of breath.

Treatment:

- CALM the patient, and remain calm yourself.
- Place in position of comfort (usually sitting or semi-sitting).
- Take a good history—find out which medications, if any, have been taken.
- Assist with the use of rescue metered dose inhaler, Albuterol, or Xopenex.
- Encourage pursed-lip breathing to create backpressure and open bronchioles.
- May do lateral chest compressions to help remove trapped air.
- Consider evacuation.

CHEST PAIN:

- There are many harmless things that cause chest pain, such as indigestion, heartburn, pulled chest wall muscles.
- Your concern with chest pain is the chance that it is cardiac.

Signs and Symptoms (cardiac):

- Left-sided, substernal chest pain that may radiate into the left arm.
- Associated with a sensation of shortness of breath.
- Associated with a cold sweat.
- Is made worse by exertion and anxiety.

Causes:

- Non-cardiac: indigestion, heartburn, pulled muscles.
- Cardiac: acute MI, angina.

Principles of Management for Suspected Cardiac Pain:

- ☑ Goal is to minimize heart effort and strain.

- ☑ Unless you are absolutely certain that the pain is not cardiac, evacuate.

- ☑ The cardiac patient should be kept at rest, as exertion will make the pain worse.

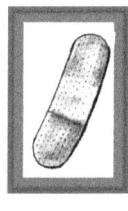

☑ Transport in a position of comfort to support breathing.

☑ Keep them calm, reassure.

☑ If you have aspirin with you, give them 1 adult (325mg) or 4 baby aspirin (unless allergic to aspirin).

☑ Get help; this patient needs to be evacuated **ASAP**.

ANAPHYLACTIC REACTION:

■ Is a severe, life-threatening allergic reaction.

Signs and Symptoms:

■ The patient usually knows if they are allergic and will tell you (but ask anyway).

■ They may have a rash—hives.

■ They may have increasing shortness of breath.

■ They may feel increasingly anxious, even terrified.

■ They may wheeze and/or have difficulty breathing or speaking.

Causes:

■ Bee stings (Hymenoptera: bees, wasps, hornets, fire ants).

■ Foods, especially peanuts or seafood.

■ Medications, e.g. penicillin.

Principles of Management:

☑ Immediately give antihistamine: Benadryl, 50mg every 4 hours for 24 hours; other antihistamines will also work.

☑ If they begin to lose their airway (SOB, wheezing), give epinephrine with an Epi-Pen or Twinject.

☑ Once able to breathe and swallow, give them the antihistamine as explained above.

☑ A second dose of epinephrine may be given if the first dose wears off before the antihistamine is absorbed.

☑ Evacuate immediately.

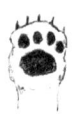

CONCUSSION DISCUSSION FOR WILDERNESS FIRST AID

Principles of Managing Head Injuries and Concussions:

Concussion refers to a blow to the head of great enough force to bruise the brain.

- Anyone who losses consciousness, regardless of how long they were unconscious, must be evacuated to definitive care.
- Anyone who has a change in level of consciousness, must be evacuated to definitive care.
  - Monitor Level Of Consciousness using the AVPU scale.
- A head injury or possible concussion, without the loss of consciousness, must be evacuated to definitive care if they:
  - Have or develop a headache.
  - Have or develop mental confusion or memory loss.
  - Have or develop any change in vision.
  - Have or develop dizziness or loss of balance.
  - Have or develop nausea with or without vomiting.
    Have or develop slurred speech or difficulty finding words.

The biggest risk to a concussion is having a second concussion within 5 days of the first.

Remember: if you suspect a head injury your "treatment" on the first aid level is to evacuate to definitive care!

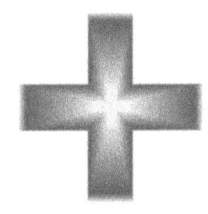

APPENDICES

SOLO—A LOOK AT WHO WE ARE

SOLO took root in the early 1970s and grew out of the vision of its founders, Dr. Frank Hubbell and Lee Frizzell (husband and wife). At that time, pre-hospital care was in its infancy, and an organized EMS system didn't exist yet in New Hampshire. The concept of providing emergency care to the sick and injured revolved around what is today referred to as the "Golden Hour." As injured skiers, climbers, and EMTs in the White Mountains of New Hampshire were being rescued, it very quickly became apparent that the skills that rescuers had learned as 'street emergency care providers did not work in a remote environment. It was obvious that people providing care in remote environments had to learn how to use skills and techniques outside the "golden hour." But, that information was not available—it had to be learned through experience. And Frank Hubbell had a great deal of experience, having been actively involved in Search and Rescue missions during college.

Frank's frustration with the lack of an appropriate "wilderness" standard led to the creation of one of the first, if not the first, organized wilderness/remote emergency medicine courses in the world. By 1975, a basic "Mountain/ Woods First Aid" course was taken on the road by Frank, and that course outline and objectives remain the foundation of SOLO's most popular course today, Wilderness First Aid. The WFA class has been adapted for a number of specialized situations like water, disaster, and expedition.

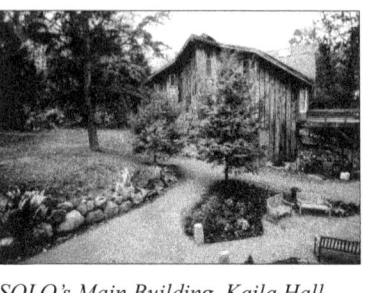

In 1976, Frank, and his wife Lee Frizzell, a trained educator, created a school in the White Mountains to develop and teach various aspects and levels of wilderness/remote/disaster medicine. They named that school SOLO, for Stonehearth Open Learning Opportunities.

SOLO's Main Building, Kaila Hall

For the next four decades SOLO continued to create more programs of varying lengths and intensity in both urban and wilderness medicine. Not only did the number of trainings at their center increase, but the numbers of sponsors grew to include colleges and universities, environmental agencies, outing clubs, rescue organizations, guiding groups, ski patrols, and many others. Pioneering immersion and experiential training techniques, SOLO was quickly recognized as always being on the cutting edge of education.

SOLO has been featured in dozens of newspaper and magazine articles as well as television programs. Many SOLO instructors regularly speak at state and national conferences.

As SOLO began to gain recognition in the emergency medical community, Frank Hubbell, previously a paramedic, went on to earn his Physician Assistant Degree before entering medical school. Not only does Frank work at SOLO teaching, helping to design curriculum and writing for the Wilderness Medicine Newsletter and other SOLO texts, he is also the senior partner and practicing physician in a large local medical practice. In addition, for the past 25 years Frank has been on NH's Medical Control Board.

SOLO founder Frank Hubbell teaching in 1980

From 2006 into the present, SOLO has enlarged its out-of-country trainings, providing courses in Tanzania, Kenya, Zambia, Turkey, Israel, Chile, Mexico, Japan, Nepal, Jordan, Costa Rica, Indonesia, Scotland, Haiti… More partnerships are being formed as programs for indigenous people have become an important focus for SOLO. Following the earthquake in Haiti, teams from SOLO made trips to that devastated nation for several months to assist in urban clinics, hospitals and rural medical centers. A specialized set of programs under the umbrella of SOLO International has been developed to better serve the needs of people in more remote areas or disaster situations.

In country we have once again begun offering advanced trainings like AEMT, ACLS, PALS, and PEARS. Our classroom has some of the most advanced multi-media equipment available.

Four decades after the official founding of SOLO, interest in wilderness/remote/disaster medicine training is still growing. Eight month-long WEMT courses are offered on our campus annually along with several dozen other programs. Hundreds of other programs continue to be offered worldwide with much of the emphasis on the disaster side of long-term care. Our campus staff now has an education department, a facilities' staff, a registrar, and several administrators who have the responsibility of dealing with a part-time list of over 250 instructors and the more than 475 courses we run annually away from the main campus. SOLO is also a formally designated American Heart Association Training Center. But to many students, the most important aspect of their SOLO experience is the all-you-can eat meals prepared by wonderful professionally trained chefs.

Since SOLO has been a licensed NH rescue unit for years, our staff and students volunteer on backcountry search and rescue missions in NH's White Mountains.

From a gathering in a living room over more than four decades, SOLO has grown into a large, diverse organization: a leader not only in medicine, but also in education and standards as well. From basic first aid—still the foundation of SOLO's purpose—we now find instructors teaching around the world. To date, SOLO has trained hundreds of thousands of people.

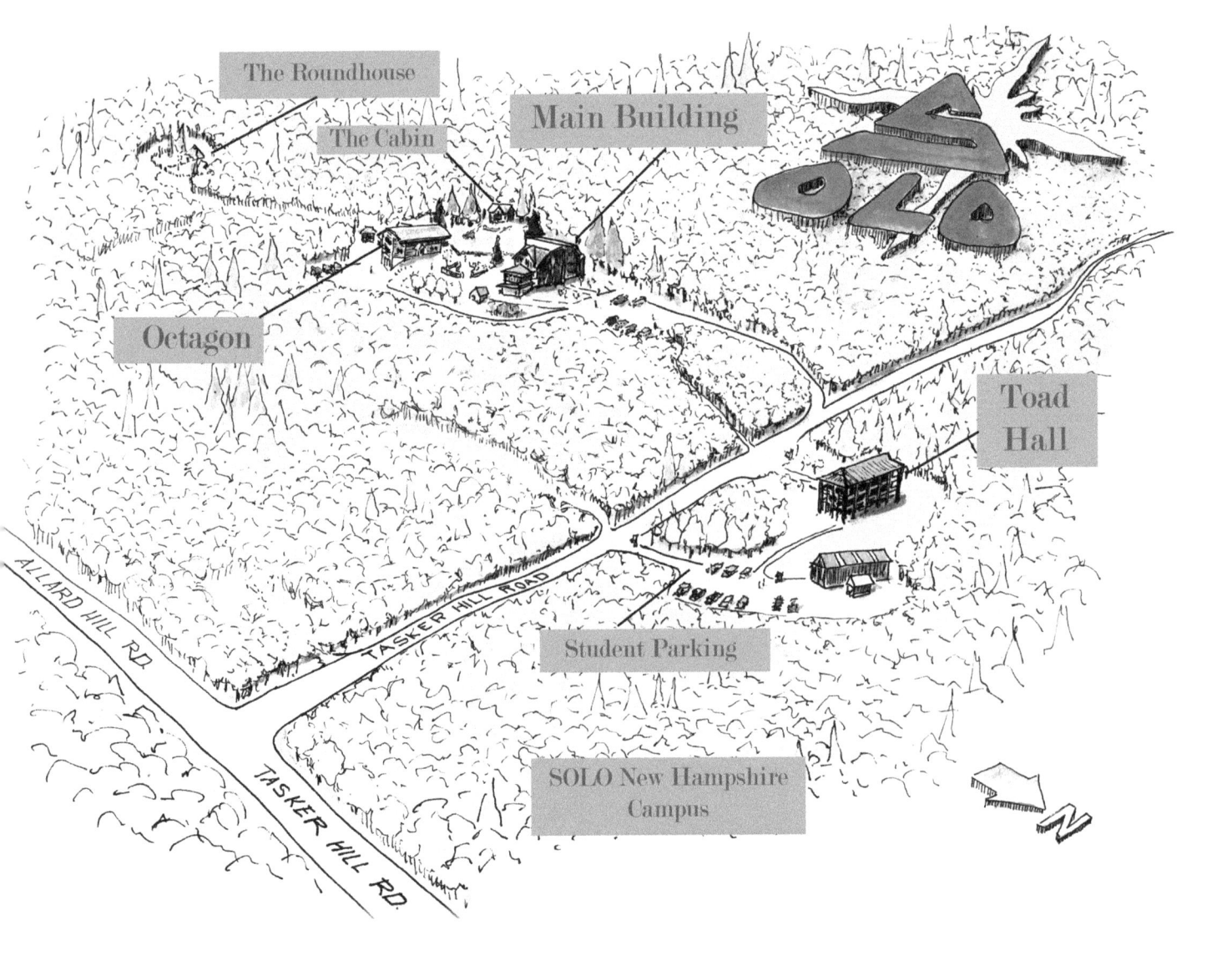

Part I quiz: Response and Assessment   **Student Name** _Saul Kaufman_

1. Which of the following are common modes of transmission of infectious disease?
   - ☐ a. Airborne by inhaling infectious particles.
   - ☐ b. Vector or insect bite.
   - ☐ c. Waterborne by drinking contaminated water.
   - ☐ d. Direct contact or bloodborne.
   - ☒ e. All of the above.

2. The purpose of the Primary Survey is all of the following except:
   - ☐ a. Find and treat all potentially life-threatening problems.
   - ☐ b. Protect from the environment.
   - ☐ c. Prevent any further injury.
   - ☒ d. Establish and monitor vital signs.

3. The Secondary Survey consists of:
   - ☐ a. Vital signs.
   - ☐ b. Patient exam.
   - ☐ c. AMPLE history.
   - ☐ d. SOAPNOTE.
   - ☒ e. All of the above.

4. All of the following AMPLE history explanations are correct except for:
   - ☐ a. A = allergies.
   - ☐ b. M = medications.
   - ☐ c. P = previous injuries or illness.
   - ☐ d. L = last in and out.
   - ☒ e. E = environmental conditions.

5. The Objective part of the SOAPnote will contain all of the following except:
   - ☐ a. Heart rate, respiratory rate and effort, & level of consciousness.
   - ☐ b. Description of locations of pain, tenderness, and injuries.
   - ☐ c. AMPLE history.
   - ☒ d. Condition of the group as a whole.

Part II quiz: Trauma: Musculoskeletal Injuries: **Student Name** _____

1. A sprain or strain can cause injury to all of the following except:
   - ☐ a. Muscle.
   - ☐ b. Tendon.
   - ☐ c. Ligament.
   - ☒ d. Bone.

2. All of the following are correct for treating a sprain except:
   - ☐ a. Rest, stop, and sit down.
   - ☐ b. Ice for vasoconstriction.
   - ☐ c. Compression with an ACE bandage.
   - ☐ d. Elevation to decrease circulation to the affected area.
   - ☒ e. Mild exercise to encourage healing.

3. Which of the following statements regarding fractures is correct?
   - ☐ a. There is typically point tenderness over the fracture site.
   - ☐ b. The patient may have felt something snap, crack, or pop.
   - ☐ c. There may be discoloration, swelling, or deformity.
   - ☐ d. There is a loss of normal function.
   - ☒ e. All are correct.

4. The most important aspect of fracture care is to:
   - ☐ a. Maintain normal function and range of motion.
   - ☒ b. Maintain circulation distal to the site of the injury.
   - ☐ c. Adjust the fracture site until there is normal sensation and movement.
   - ☐ d. Splint the fracture exactly the way you found it.

5. The reason to straighten out an angulated fracture is to:
   - ☐ a. Make it easier to splint.
   - ☐ b. Place the injury in a more comfortable position.
   - ☒ c. Establish and maintain circulation.
   - ☐ d. Place it in the proper position for healing.

6. Splints should be monitored every 15 minutes to:
   - ☐ a. Make sure that the splint is still tight and snug.
   - ☐ b. Make sure the fracture is in the proper position.
   - ☐ c. Make sure the extremity is staying cool so that it will not swell.
   - ☒ d. Make sure there is circulation distal to the fracture.

7. Which of the following statements is incorrect regarding spinal injuries?
   - ☐ a. The patient must by sober and oriented x 3 to "clear" the spine.
   - ☐ b. The patient should be free of distracting injuries at the time of the exam.
   - ☒ c. If they fell more than twice their height, you must treat for a back injury.
   - ☐ d. You can move the patient from position of injury to position of function.

Part III quiz: Environmental Emergencies   **Student Name** _____

1. Circle True or False in regard to the following statements about hypothermia:
   (T)/ F Hypothermia is most commonly associated with cold, wet, windy conditions.
   (T)/ F Humans are designed to lose heat when wet.
   T /(F) Hypothermia has little or no effect on the human brain.
   (T)/ F Humans burn glucose as a fuel to help maintain body temperature.
   (T)/ F Shivering is involuntary muscular contractions that produce heat.
   T (F) Shivering does NOT impair other physical activity.
   (T)/ F Conscious hypothermia victims need water and glucose.
   T (F) Never expose and dry off a wet hypothermia patient.

2. Which of the following is incorrect regarding frostbite?
   ☐ a. Superficial frostbite can be field rewarmed with skin-to-skin contact.
   ☐ b. Deep frostbite should not be field rewarmed, but should be protected from further damage.
   ☐ c. Refreezing recently thawed frostbite will cause a much worse injury.
   ☒ d. It is preferable to use hot air to thaw frostbitten hands.

3. Which of the following is correct regarding heat stroke?
   ☐ a. Heat stroke is a minor injury associated with dehydration and salt depletion.
   ☐ b. Heat stroke is self-correcting and does not require treatment.
   ☒ c. Heat stroke patients need to be aggressively cooled with water.
   ☐ d. Heat stroke is rarely associated with dehydration.

4. When someone is sent out to get help, all of the following are true except:
   ☐ a. Keep everyone busy, and keep everyone warm and dry.
   ☐ b. Build a bivouac to protect the patient and everyone else in the group.
   ☐ c. Build a fire or light a stove to make something warm to drink.
   ☒ d. Send someone out for help every 1 – 2 hours until help arrives.

Part IV quiz: Soft Tissue Injuries and Critical Care   **Student Name** _____

1. All of the following statements are correct except:
   ☒ a. Blood is sterile and harmless to others exposed to it.
   ☐ b. Arteries are under pressure, and although rare, spurt blood when cut.
   ☐ c. Veins are low pressure and drain blood when cut.
   ☐ d. Capillaries are very small and low pressure; they ooze or seep when cut.
   ☐ e. Veins are commonly injured because they can be just under the skin.

2. All of the following statements about controlling bleeding are correct except:
   ☐ a. Pressure directly over the wound is the most effective way to control bleeding.
   ☐ b. If direct pressure is not enough, you can also elevate the wound.
   ☐ c. Pressure dressings are very effective but should only be used for about 10 minutes.
   ☒ d. Never remove a dressing once it has been placed on the wound.
   ☐ e. In extreme cases direct digital pressure can be applied directly to an open spurting artery.

3. All of the following are signs or symptoms of a localized tissue infection except:
   ☐ a. The area is red (rubor).
   ☐ b. The area is warm to the touch (calor).
   ☐ c. The area is swollen (tumor).
   ☐ d. The area is tender to the touch (dolor).
   ☒ e. The area is red but not warm to the touch.

4. Please answer True or False about severe potentially life-threatening tissue infections:
   Ⓣ/ F   There can be a collection of pus or other drainage coming from the wound.
   Ⓣ/ F   There may be red streaks running proximally from the infection site.
   Ⓣ/ F   There may be swollen tender lymph nodes proximal to the infection site.
   Ⓣ F   The patient may have fever and chills.
   Ⓣ F   Wound infections can be prevented by proper cleaning and bandaging.
   T /Ⓕ   Wounds associated with impairment of circulation, sensation, or movement
           do not need to be immediately evacuated; they can wait 2 – 3 days.

5. Which statement is incorrect in regard to impaled objects?
   ☒ a. Never remove impaled objects.
   ☐ b. Remove impaled objects that are in an extremity.
   ☐ c. Remove metal impaled objects in a cold environment.
   ☐ d. Do not remove impaled objects in the skull, neck, chest, or abdomen.

6. Which of the following statements is incorrect about thermal burns.
   ☐ a. Immediately cold soak the burn area with cold water for about 15 minutes.
   ☒ b. Superficial burns rarely cause very much pain.
   ☐ c. Deep burns have minimal pain due to nerve destruction in the skin.
   ☐ d. All deep burns patients need to be hydrated and evacuated.

— NOTES —

SOAPNOTE

Subjective: age, sex, mechanism of injury (MOI), chief complaint(C/C): _____

_____

_____

_____

_____

Objective: vital signs, patient exam, AMPLE history:

Vital Signs

TIME					
LOC oriented x ?					
RR & effort					
HR & effort					
Skin C, T, M					

Patient Exam: Describe locations of pain, tenderness & injuries:

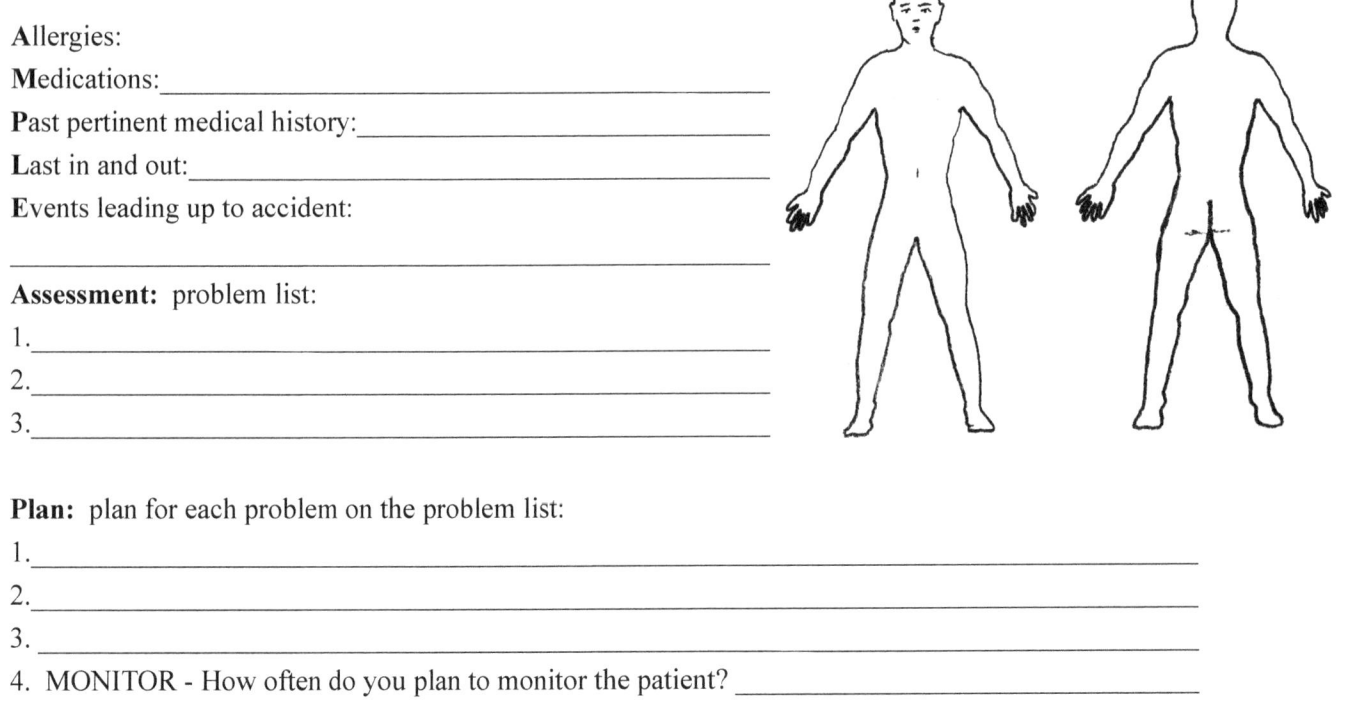

Allergies:

Medications:_____

Past pertinent medical history:_____

Last in and out:_____

Events leading up to accident:

_____

Assessment: problem list:

1._____

2._____

3._____

Plan: plan for each problem on the problem list:

1._____

2._____

3. _____

4. MONITOR - How often do you plan to monitor the patient? _____

SOAPNOTE

Subjective: age, sex, mechanism of injury (MOI), chief complaint(C/C): _____

_____

_____

_____

_____

Objective: vital signs, patient exam, AMPLE history:

Vital Signs

TIME					
LOC oriented x ?					
RR & effort					
HR & effort					
Skin C, T, M					

Patient Exam: Describe locations of pain, tenderness & injuries:

Allergies:

Medications:_____

Past pertinent medical history:_____

Last in and out:_____

Events leading up to accident:

_____

Assessment: problem list:

1._____

2._____

3._____

Plan: plan for each problem on the problem list:

1._____

2._____

3. _____

4. MONITOR - How often do you plan to monitor the patient? _____

SOAPNOTE

Subjective: age, sex, mechanism of injury (MOI), chief complaint(C/C): _____

_____

_____

_____

_____

Objective: vital signs, patient exam, AMPLE history:

Vital Signs

TIME					
LOC oriented x ?					
RR & effort					
HR & effort					
Skin C, T, M					

Patient Exam: Describe locations of pain, tenderness & injuries:

Allergies:

Medications:_____

Past pertinent medical history:_____

Last in and out:_____

Events leading up to accident:

_____

Assessment: problem list:

1._____

2._____

3._____

Plan: plan for each problem on the problem list:

1._____

2._____

3. _____

4. MONITOR - How often do you plan to monitor the patient? _____

Upon successful completion of this course you will be able to perform:

Patient Assessment System and Critical Care

Scene Survey – Scene Safety

Primary Survey – Life Threats

Secondary Survey

Rescue Survey

Shock – recognition and treatment of shock

Trauma: Musculoskeletal Injuries – Recognition and Treatment of:

Sprain and strains and Fractures

Upper extremity injuries:

Sling and Swathe

Forearm/wrist splint

Lower leg and knee injuries:

Lower leg and knee splints

Soft Tissue and Medical Emergencies:

Control of Bleeding

Long-term wound care

Bandaging skills:

Scalp bandage

Temporal bandage

Arm sling and swathe

Shoulder and hip bandage

Knee bandage

Sprained ankle bandage

Thermal burn care

Blister care

Medical Emergencies – Recognition and Management of:

Change in Level Of Consciousness

Chest pain

Shortness of breath and Asthma

Anaphylaxis

Environmental Emergencies – Recognition and Management of:

Hypothermia and Frostbite

Heat Stroke, Heat Exhaustion, and dehydration

North American Bites and Stings

Lightning

Bivouac and Survival Skills

SOLO
Stonehearth Open Learning Opportunities

We hope that you enjoy your SOLO course. SOLO is the nation's leader in wilderness medicine education with hundreds of thousands of students attending courses since 1976. SOLO has been instrumental in the development of Wilderness First Aid, Wilderness First Responder, and Wilderness EMT curricula. Our campus, perched

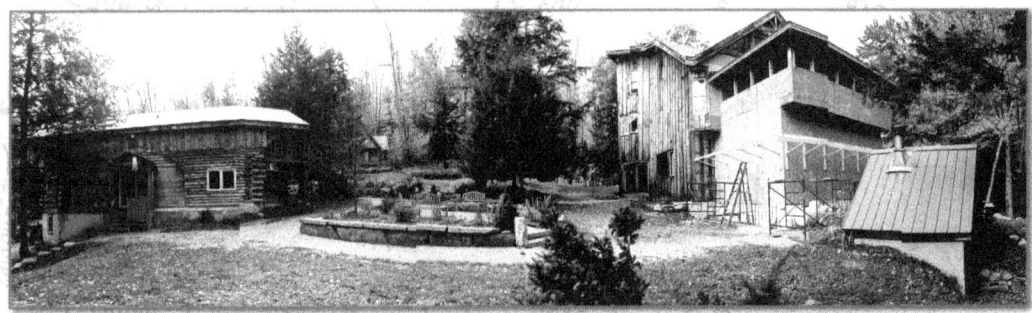

on 300 acres in the heart of New Hampshire's White Mountains, is a unique teaching facility made up of our three-story Main Building, a 30-person dorm, dining hall, and other facilities. Find out more about SOLO by visiting soloschools.com. We hope you decide to continue your wilderness medicine education by attending one of our other programs.

SOLO, PO Box 3150, Conway, NH 03818 • 603-447-6711

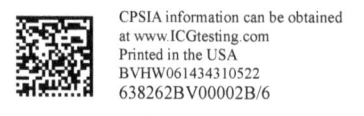